HEAL YOUR HEART
with **Wine** *and* **Chocolate**

...AND 99 OTHER WAYS WOMEN
CAN PROTECT THEIR HEARTS

HEAL YOUR HEART
with **Wine** *and* **Chocolate**

...AND 99 OTHER WAYS WOMEN CAN PROTECT THEIR HEARTS

DEBORA YOST

Foreword by **NANCY LOVING**
Executive Director, WomenHeart: The National Coalition for Women with Heart Disease

STC Healthy Living
Stewart, Tabori & Chang • New York

Excerpts of individual experiences were reprinted with permission from *Stories from the Heart: Women Heart Patients Describe Their Disease, Treatment and Recovery*, compiled and arranged by Anastasis Roussos and Melissa Lausin. Copyright © 2003 by WomenHeart: National Coalition for Women with Heart Disease.

Published in 2006 by
Stewart, Tabori & Chang
115 West 18th Street
New York, NY 10011
www.abramsbooks.com

Printed in USA
Designed by Wendy Palitz & Neil Egan

Library of Congress Cataloging-in-Publication Data

Yost, Debora.
  Heal your heart with wine and chocolate: ...and 99 other ways women
  can protect their hearts / by Debora Yost; foreword by Nancy Loving.
     p.   cm.
  Includes bibliographical references.
  ISBN 1-58479-437-2
1. Heart—Diseases—Diet therapy. 2. Heart—Diseases—Prevention.
2.
RC684.D5Y67 2006
616.1'205—dc22
                                      2005023279

The text of this book was composed in HTF Gotham and Caecilia.

10 9 8 7 6 5 4 3 2 1
First Printing

Stewart, Tabori & Chang is an imprint of

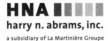

HNA ▮▮▮▮▮
harry n. abrams, inc.
a subsidiary of La Martinière Groupe

For Nick

Contents

> *"Good health and good sense are two of life's greatest blessings."* —Publius Syrus, 42 B.C. Maxim 827

· Acknowledgments ·

The idea for *Heal Your Heart with Wine and Chocolate* actually came about 8 years ago when I was working with the editor of a women's magazine to develop cover lines for future issues. Sometimes in the journalism business, a good headline develops a story idea, instead of the other way around.

In this case, it was a headline that didn't pan out. The research on the health benefits of chocolate was promising, but unproven, and doctors were reluctant to go on record recommending anything alcoholic as healthy. Off the record, the physicians were candidly optimistic about the health benefits of moderate drinking. But the idea of telling patients to drink wine, even backed with the caveat that it should be limited to a glass a day, just seemed too extreme at the time.

Then a few years ago, a close friend of mine had a heart attack. I remember getting the call: "You aren't going to believe this, but Kathy had a heart attack. Carl [her husband] got her to the hospital in time—thank God he wasn't out of town!"

Kathy, now living a healthy and active life, was 54 when it happened.

Even though I've been a health writer and health book editor throughout most of my career, I was stunned: At 54—a woman? Yes, I did know that heart disease was the number-one cause of death among women, but I will confess that I was among the 87 percent of all women in the United States who believed it was not a threat to me—or to my friends. I knew heart disease was largely preventable and not a natural part of aging. I knew there are lots of things that are bad for the heart—certain foods, lack of exercise, and that hard-to-measure and hard-to-define menace called stress.

Lots of things we shouldn't do, lots of things we shouldn't eat—how's that for a gloomy future? I thought of Kathy's long list of "can't haves" and "can't do's," and I figured there had to be a better, more positive way to look to the future.

So, I started to do research for something that might cheer Kathy up, and that line about "heal your heart with wine and chocolate" popped into my mind. By this time, the scientific research was more concrete—and positive. I called R. Curtis Ellison, M.D., one of America's leading heart researchers and Chief of Preventive Medicine and Epidemiology at Boston University School of Medicine. He has done much of the research on wine and, at the time, was concluding a major study on chocolate. He confirmed my suspicion that it was now "safe" to say that drinking wine and eating chocolate, in moderation and as part of an overall healthy lifestyle, can be good for the heart.

Overall healthy lifestyle . . . that is the key to a healthy heart. So I thought: what if the things required to live a healthy lifestyle were put in terms of good things you can do? What other healthy habits would have a special appeal to women? The more I researched, the more those "things" started to add up. This wasn't an idea for a magazine article; there was enough to fill an entire book.

As part of my research, I was tapping into a web site called WomenHeart.org, which is the online engine for the National Coalition for Women with Heart Disease. I called Nancy Loving, the Executive Director and co-founder, and—no surprise—found her to be exceptionally encouraging about the book idea. Over the 9 months I spent researching and writing, Nancy was very helpful in giving me leads and introductions to key heart specialists whom I could interview for this book. She offered excellent advice on how to shape the book, especially in terms of the gender disparities that exist in the way women and men accumulate risk factors, experience heart disease and heart attacks, and how they deal with the recovery stage of a heart attack. I am grateful to her and also to the members of WomenHeart who shared personal anecdotes from the book, *Stories from the Heart*. They are quoted throughout this book.

I thank Sharonne N. Hayes, M.D., Director of the Women's Health Clinic at Mayo Clinic in Rochester, Minnesota, for reviewing this book for medical accuracy and helping me translate technical terms and medical procedures into everyday language. Any errors, however, are all mine.

I also thank author Wayne M. Sotile, Ph.D., Director of Psychological Services at Wake Forest University Healthy Exercise and Lifestyle Programs, for graciously sharing his unique experiences as an expert on the emotional issues that confront women with heart disease.

My sincere gratitude goes to Leslie Stoker, my editor and publisher at Stewart, Tabori & Chang, for her smart suggestions and unbelievable patience.

I would also like to give special mention to some of the many others who helped with this book: Lisa Andruscavage, copy editor, friend, and former colleague; Wendy Palitz and Neil Egan, who designed the book, and STC's Galen Smith, Andrea Glickson, Kim Tyner, Marianne Patela, Kate Norment, Jennifer Levesque, and Marisa Bulzone, for giving me help and encouragement.

Take It One Tip at a Time

When I had a heart attack at age 48, I didn't know women could have heart attacks. To be truthful, I didn't even know women could get heart disease. Apparently, my doctors didn't know either. Our collective ignorance nearly killed me.

Like so many younger women, I had only seen obstetrician/gynecologists for all my health care needs since I was in college. None of them ever mentioned "heart disease" to me, even though they knew my father and other relatives had all died young of heart attacks. But my mother had breast cancer in her late fifties, so I—and my doctors—were focused on my annual mammograms.

What we didn't pay attention to was my cholesterol, which had not been tested for at least 10 years. It was an astonishing 313 when I had the heart attack! Neither were we paying attention to my stress levels as a busy executive and single mother of two teenagers—it was off the charts. I was very stressed, always tired, smoked socially, did not take time for exercise, and doing a very poor job of taking care of myself. I was a walking heart attack waiting to happen.

When I did have the heart attack, I had strange symptoms—upper back pressure, lightheadedness, and nausea. I thought maybe I had the flu or food poisoning. But when I began to feel faint, I asked my daughter to drive me to the nearest emergency room. Luckily, I was seen by an ER doctor who quickly recognized my symptoms as heart-related and diagnosed a heart attack. He then gave me a "clot buster" medicine that immediately dissolved the clot that was causing the attack. My symptoms instantly disappeared, so I told him I had a conference call that I needed to be on in two hours and asked if could I be discharged by then. "We need to talk..." was his wary reply.

I was admitted to the Intensive Care Unit, and then discharged from the hospital several days later. No one ever did come in to talk to me, but while I was sleeping someone left me brochures about cholesterol, blood pressure, and eating more vegetables. I was not referred to cardiac rehabilitation and returned to work part-time in two weeks.

The heart attack was traumatic because I did not realize I was at risk in spite of my family history, nor did I recognize my symptoms as heart-related. Turns out, my symptoms were very typical of those many women experience. The real trauma came, however, as a result of the social isolation I felt during my so-called recovery. I could not find a support group anywhere, except ones filled with older men who'd survived bypass surgery. I pleaded with my cardiologists to connect me with other young women heart attack survivors but they could not or chose not to help. I believe they just didn't understand why it was important to me. This led me to become ever more isolated and anxious. I became clinically depressed.

When I finally connected with several women heart attack survivors in 1997, I learned that their heart attacks had been misdiagnosed in the ER and they had received very poor medical treatment. We became very angry at this inexcusable state of affairs, outraged by the collective ignorance, and vowed to never let what happened to us happen to one other woman. We then formed WomenHeart:

the National Coalition for Women with Heart Disease and officially opened for business in April 2000.

WomenHeart is a mission-driven organization. We aim to improve the quality of life and health care for the 8 million American women who are living with heart disease, and to advocate on their behalf. We believe every woman has the right to early detection, accurate diagnosis, and proper treatment of her heart disease. We are also working hard to eliminate the misdiagnosis, delayed diagnosis, mistreatment, and under-treatment that so many women with heart disease encounter within the health-care system, as well as its gender-based disparities in cardiac research studies and access to quality treatments.

Most of all, WomenHeart is committed to prevention. We are convinced that the best strategy is to educate women to take charge of their heart health, to understand their cardiac risk factors, and help them take the correct actions to reduce them. We also believe in the power of knowledge about which effective actions will best help women live longer and more heart healthy lives—a benefit for themselves, for sure, but also for their families who depend upon them.

That's where the 101 tips outlined in this book come in. They are your roadmap to a happier and healthy life—one filled with energy and calm, friendship and health. The most important message is that you give yourself permission to take much better care of yourself—to make sure you take time for yourself every day, and also make time to spend with your family and women friends. It's not a question of being selfish—it's a question of saving your life and preventing premature disability or death.

Do not try to implement all 101 tips at once. It would be too overwhelming and make you discouraged—a recipe for certain failure! Instead, savor them slowly, trying one or two at a time. If you can make a commitment to incorporate one tip into your life each week, at the end of one year you will have made a dramatic change in the way you care for yourself and your body. We all know how hard it is to change our behavior, so be patient and kind to yourself. But understand one thing for certain: it's your heart and only you can take good care of it! Enjoy.

Nancy Loving

Executive Director and co-founder
WomenHeart: The National Coalition
for Women with Heart Disease

December 2005

1 What **Women** Need to Know

In affairs of the heart, songwriters say, women are the last to know. The same can be said for diseases of the heart. In fact, this year, 500,000 American women will find out about it the hard way: They'll have a heart attack.

Here's the hard heart truth: More women will die from cardiovascular disease this year than from the next 15 causes of death combined. It is a stunning reality that is finally making physicians, researchers, and women themselves take notice.

Today, more women than ever before—46 percent—are aware that heart disease is their number one killer. Yet only 13 percent of women consider heart disease as a major threat to their personal health. It is an error in judgment with life-and-death consequences, especially when you consider that heart disease kills six times as many women as breast cancer and twice as many women than all forms of cancer combined.

This disconnect can be attributed, at least in part, to the long-held belief that heart disease is a "man's disease." It is the most enduring myth in modern medicine. Consider:

- ♥ Women have as many heart attacks as men but we are more likely to die from one.

- ♥ More women than men die of heart disease each year.

- ♥ 38 percent of women, compared to 25 percent of men, die within 1 year of a first heart attack.

- ♥ Among the survivors, 35 percent of women, compared to 18 percent of men, will have a second heart attack within 6 years.

- ♥ Twice as many women as men will end up disabled as a result of heart disease.

- ♥ Women are twice as likely as men to die after having bypass surgery.

What Kills Women

Cardiovascular disease—heart attack, heart disease, and stroke—kills more women each year than all of these causes combined:

- All forms of cancer
- Respiratory illnesses
- Alzheimer's disease
- Diabetes
- Accidents
- Liver disease
- Kidney disease
- Flu and pneumonia
- Blood poisoning

Surprised? Most women are. Even more revealing is the fact that heart-related deaths, thanks mostly to advances in medicine and medical science, actually have gone down over the last 40 years in both men and women. But the decline has been slower in women, especially among women of color. And nonfatal heart attacks in women have actually gone up 36 percent compared to a 6 percent drop in men.

So, what's going on?

For one, virtually all the medical research into heart disease causes and cures over the past several decades has been done on men. Studies that included women did so in limited number. Meanwhile, the heart disease "norm" in hospitals, medical schools, and doctors' offices has been modeled after a 165-pound man and a male lifestyle. But, as Neica Goldberg, M.D., so appropriately notes, "women are not small men"—in fact, she wrote a book about women and heart disese called *Women Are Not Small Men*.

Second, it has only been in recent years that medical science started to recognize that heart attacks often occur differently in women than in men, an acknowledgement that at least in part helps explain why:

- ♥ 35 percent of first heart attacks in women go unreported or unnoticed.

- ♥ It takes medical emergency teams longer to react to symptoms of a heart attack in women than in men.

Third, even though men and women share equally in the disease, women get less-aggressive treatment:

- ♥ More women than men die of heart disease, yet only one-third of invasive life-saving treatments such as stents and bypass surgery, and 20 percent of implantable defibrillators, are recommended for women.

♥ Women are less likely than men to be given medications such as beta-blockers or even aspirin after a heart attack.

♥ Five times as many men as women are sent to cardiac rehabilitation after a heart attack.

And ponder this: A 50-year-old woman hospitalized for a heart attack is twice as likely as a male heart attack victim the same age to never make it out of the hospital alive.

A MEDICAL MYTH

"I called 911 when I had severe heartburn and back pain, sweating, and shortness of breath. The emergency room doctor discharged me and said to stop and buy a bottle of Mylanta on my way home. Twelve hours later, my mother found me on the floor, nearly unconscious and having a full-blown heart attack." —Susan, age 41

It is not that heart specialists have intentionally been ignoring women. By medical training and practice, the heart had always been viewed as gender-neutral. Traditionally, women were considered virtually immune to heart disease until after the age of menopause when heart-protecting estrogen goes into a dramatic decline. Women under the age of 60 or so simply didn't get heart attacks. If they did, it was considered an anomaly or written off as bad genes.

Medicine now knows differently. Heart disease is an equal-opportunity aggressor; it just announces its presence about 10 years earlier in men. By age 40, a woman's lifetime risk of developing heart disease is only 32 percent compared to 49 percent for men. The gap, however, rapidly narrows, then closes with advancing years. By age 55, the number of women with heart disease is double that of younger women, and after age 65, it rises twelvefold.

Doctors in the Dark

If you're among the women who did not realize that heart disease kills more women every year than men, you are in esteemed, albeit startling, company—1 out of 5 doctors.

At least they didn't know this as recently as February 2005 when researchers from various heart centers in the United States released the results of a random online study that set out to evaluate physician adherence to new cardiovascular disease guidelines. Among the 500 physicians surveyed—100 cardiologists, 100 obstetricians/gynecologists, and 300 primary care physicians—fewer than 1 in 5 physicians knew that more women than men die each year from cardiovascular disease, reported the researchers.

The study also found that women who "were considered at intermediate risk for heart disease were significantly more likely to be assigned to a lower-risk category by primary care physicians than men with identical risk profiles."

The assessments were based on answers to questionnaires filled out by the doctors.

Heart disease isn't something that comes on suddenly like a cold or the flu. It develops slowly and silently, manifesting itself over years and starting, in some instances, as early as childhood. It is so sneaky that 64 percent of women (compared to 50 percent of men) who die suddenly from a heart attack had no known symptoms.

By the middle years of 45 to 54, one-third of all women have heart disease—and most won't even realize it until it makes its presence known by a heart attack. Unfortunately for us, the warning signs and even an attack itself can strike a woman uncharacteristically—that is to say, not the way doctors have been trained to think "heart attack". The most common symptom of a heart attack in both men and women is some kind of pain and/or pressure and discomfort in the chest. In women, however, the pain is not always severe or even the most prominent symptom. Women can experience other, more subtle flu-like symptoms like back and neck pain, indigestion, and nausea—signs that can keep them waiting too long for help in an emergency room or, even worse, sent home with medicine for indigestion. No matter what the symptoms, however, the reality of having a heart attack leaves nearly all women stunned, because they never saw it coming.

TWO HEARTS ARE NOT AS ONE

"I knew something was wrong, especially the way I got breathless at the gym. My doctor said it was my asthma acting up. The morning after I had a heart attack that almost killed me, my doctor called and said, 'What happened?' I said to her, 'You tell me!' " —Kathy, age 54

Women's Unmanly Symptoms

Intense pain and tightness in the chest, shortness of breath, and pain that radiates down the left arm are classic symptoms of a heart attack. In women, however, chest pain is often less severe. Women also can experience "unclassic" symptoms like:

- Discomfort similar to indigestion
- Back and neck pain
- Unrelenting fatigue
- Pressure in the upper abdomen

These symptoms have and can cause a misdiagnosis or a delay in diagnosis in women. Like a heart attack, the symptoms of heart *disease* also can be more subtle in women than in men, says Sharonne N. Hayes, M.D., Director of the Women's Heart Clinic at Mayo Clinic in Rochester, Minnesota. It is why so many women who have a heart attack don't even know they had heart disease.

"Any kind of symptom that is new, like breathlessness after normal activity or unexplained dizziness, should not be ignored because it may be a sign of heart disease," says Dr. Hayes. "Report it to your doctor."

Heart attacks do not discriminate between men and women. A heart attack occurs when a plaque-filled artery suddenly closes, blocking blood from getting to a portion of the heart muscle. Heart *disease*, however, can progress quite differently in men and women. Often, the complaints that bring women to the doctor's office are caused by blockages in smaller, less-flexible vessels, rather than the major arteries, where blockages typically are found in men. The major arteries in women are likely to have only mild or more diffuse blockages.

This is significant because blockage in the major arteries is what doctors look for during a coronary angiography, a procedure in which dye is injected into the heart arteries to detect blockage. When the test is done on a woman with suspected heart disease, the large vessels can look clear. The diagnosis: *Whatever it is, it isn't heart disease.* So, home she goes, with an unsure diagnosis at best.

This is not a rare occurrence. A review of procedures done on 33,202 men and women admitted with symptoms of a heart attack to 100 hospitals in 14 countries cited a close-to-normal electrocardiogram as a prime reason why so many women who are admitted to the hospital for a heart attack are discharged without a firm diagnosis or with less aggressive drug-therapy treatment. This same investigation showed that heart attack was ruled out even in instances where a woman's blood enzyme test was identical to the results doctors used to conclude that a heart attack did indeed take place in a man.

Other studies have found similar incongruities in the treatment women receive in hospitals. In general, studies show that women experienced longer delays between diagnosis and treatment and were given less-aggressive treatment, especially if the woman was older. In one study in Canada, a clot-dissolving drug that is supposed to be given to all patients admitted for a heart attack was not always administered to women. And in Michigan, emergency vehicles transporting women with symptoms of a heart attack arrived on average 20 minutes later than ambulances responding to men in distress.

When it comes to operating room procedures, the statistics are even more ominous. Women get fewer invasive procedures than men. For example, in one recent year, 4 million surgical procedures, from angioplasty to coronary bypass surgery, were done on men compared to 2.8 million on women. Out of 571,000 bypass surgeries, only 182,000 were done on women. Yet, statistics also show that women who get the procedures do better than women who do not receive the procedures.

It all comes down to this very discomforting reality: The in-hospital death rate after a heart attack is higher in women than in men, and highest in women over age 60.

MAKING PROGRESS

"I am fortunate my physician took my symptoms seriously. I was the one who didn't want to believe it was cardiac-related. I was the one looking for other excuses. I was truly in denial." —Patty, age 49

During the last few years, a lot of progress has been made in understanding that women are not like men when it comes to heart disease, thanks to the National Heart, Lung and Blood Institute's "Heart Truth" campaign, WomenHeart: the National Coalition for Women with Heart Disease, other women's health advocacy groups, and the American Heart Association. Many hospitals now have programs or diagnostic centers devoted exclusively to women and heart disease, such as the Women's Heart Clinic at Mayo Clinic in Rochester, Minnesota. New hospital practice guidelines have been issued for nurses and doctors to recognize a woman's unique symptoms, and new diagnostic tools are being used that can better identify blockages in female hearts.

Heart research studies now include more women, though women still only represent about 25 percent of participants. And in 2005, for the first time, the American Heart Association's Second International Conference on Women, Heart Disease, and Stroke (notice it was only the second) announced that women hospitalized for heart attacks are now just as likely as men to be discharged on the same recommended drug therapy as men. The AHA viewed this as progress.

Progress is exactly what is needed to correct the misconceptions that have unintentionally put women in peril. Hopefully, progress will be swift. It is comforting to know that measures are now in place and doctors and nurses are getting the training to act on a woman's nonclassic complaints when she winds up in the emergency room. The tougher goal is keeping us out of the emergency room in the first place by reducing our risk of heart disease. We can't depend on others for that. We have to make that happen ourselves, for here's another hard heart truth: Heart disease does not have to be a woman's biggest enemy. Studies show that every woman has the personal power to significantly reduce her risk of heart disease simply by the way she chooses to lead her daily life.

WHAT WE NEED TO DO

"After my heart attack, I learned to be my own best health advocate. I really want to know what diagnostic tests are available and how they can help me." —Kathleen, age 46

In the year 2000, only 6 percent of women considered heart disease their number one personal health threat. Today that number is a little more than double. That's hardly enough. We all need to recognize that heart disease is a personal threat—not something that happens to somebody else. In this, we have a long way to go. We need some self-education, too. Though 90 percent of women know that a healthy diet, exercise, and not smoking help prevent heart disease, the majority is uncertain as to the specific measures they can take. Research has found the greatest lack of knowledge among women 45 and younger. Considering that one in eight women in this age group will have a heart attack at some time in her life, this is a concern we need to do something about.

And that is the purpose of this book. During my 25 years as a health journalist, I've heard women grousing that heart-healthy practices are a list of "have nots." That is not quite true, because even the worst heart-offending practices, like eating fast food, are not harmful as long as you view them as a rare treat.

This is not a book of have nots. It is a book of "must haves." Many heart-smart choices are things women enjoy, like having a glass of wine. Some are things we crave, like a little chocolate. Some are a treat, like escaping for a weekend trip to the mountains. Many are things women just don't give themselves permission to do, like having a massage or hiring a babysitter just to spend some quiet time alone.

Consider this book a permission slip. The 101 little things recommended in the pages that follow can take you a long way toward dramatically reducing your risk of heart disease.

And speaking of risk, if heart disease is different in men and women, it is correct to assume that we accumulate many of these risks in different ways. Medical science now knows that what is considered normal for one sex is not necessarily the same for the other. Men and women can even be different in some of the approaches they should take to protect their hearts.

All 101 tips in this book are based on medical research that shows a measurable benefit. All are female-friendly and, where possible, results are reported for women exclusively. The place to begin your personal heart-protection program is in understanding women's risk factors and figuring out your own. The good news is that you have the power to help keep your heart healthy. As you read on, you'll find out why.

2 Know Your **Risk**

The first thing every woman should do to protect her heart is to be aware of the unhealthy habits that put her in jeopardy. The second thing is to do something about them. The fact that we have the ability to significantly reduce our risk of heart disease should be a powerful incentive to change the lifestyle habits that can keep us from living a long and healthy life.

The evidence is overwhelming: The way we live our lives has a greater impact on preventing heart problems than any other disease. If you've already had a heart attack, studies show that a combination of lifestyle changes is more powerful than any one alone in preventing a second one.

The American Heart Association (AHA) and the National Institutes of Health emphasize five major risks that lead to heart disease: smoking, obesity, diabetes, high blood pressure, and high cholesterol.

We have the power to control all of them, but success depends on our level of commitment.

Along with the information that men and women experience heart disease differently is the knowledge that gender plays a part in how we develop risks and what we can do to prevent them. Being female works for and against us, depending on the risk. But here's the most important thing: No matter what your age, it is not too late to protect your heart.

START NOW

"I knew life was short. Now I understand that an ignored symptom here, a hurried doctor there, being too timid to question authority—any of them could have erased me from this life like a pencil line from paper. I deserve more than that." — Laurie, who received two stents to open major artery blockage on her 48th birthday

Is your doctor close to your heart?

If you do not get an annual physical exam beyond the routine ritual that takes place in your gynecologist's office, you should. "Old-time medical exams are being replaced by age-related health assessments and are a big part of preventive care," says Bob Sheff, M.D., author of *The Medical Mentor* and a physician who has spent much of his career as the top administrator for a health maintenance organization (HMO). If you depend on your gynecologist as your primary-care physician, you may be missing out on some of the important procedures that involve your heart.

"Many gynecologists are uncomfortable providing preventive care beyond their specialty," says Dr. Sheff. "It might happen by default if a woman is using her gynecologist for primary care. But it is in a woman's best interest to also have a primary-care physician in addition to a gynecologist."

Your gynecologist is concerned about you, so don't hesitate to ask for a referral to a doctor who can be your whole-health provider. This could be a family practitioner or internist.

Once you've found the right physician, you need to get a complete and understandable assessment of your health. Here is what Dr. Sheff says you should do.

Tip 1: **Have a Heart-to-Heart with Your Doctor**

This should begin with your physician probing for a family history of heart disease. If she doesn't ask, then offer the information (but consider it a red flag if she doesn't ask). It is information essential to your health care. Dr. Sheff recommends that you arrive at the doctor's office with your questions and concerns written down so you don't forget anything important. If your doctor acts indifferent or won't give you adequate time for a discussion, get another doctor.

Get the details. When your doctor, or more likely the nurse, calls with test results, ask for specifics. Do not accept reports like "everything is normal" or "your cholesterol is a little high but it's nothing to be concerned about yet." Nurses often don't get into details because they are very busy or because they assume that you won't understand how to interpret the results. Do not settle for anything less than a complete explanation. Take notes and ask questions. And don't hesitate to say, "Please slow down, you're talking too fast."

Start a record. Ask that the report be sent to you. If the nurse seems annoyed because she already explained it all on the phone, well, too bad. Don't back off. You should be no more intimidated by medical people than you are by the clerks in the checkout line at the supermarket. You can offer to pick up the report, but if the nurse is doing her job, she'll gladly drop it in the mail.

Remember, you didn't make this request just to get back at a doctor for keeping you waiting too long in a cold room wearing nothing but a paper robe. The exam results and any impressions you formed during the visit could be very important in the future. File them away in a place that you'll remember.

Be sure. If you are left with one scintilla of concern about your heart health, ask for a referral to a cardiologist.

THE HIGH FIVE

"I realized something was wrong with my body when my blood pressure would not measure on the drugstore blood pressure machine!" — Helen, diagnosed with heart disease at age 70

There is one universal heart fact common to all ages, genders, races, and countries of origin: The likelihood of a heart attack rises proportionally with the accumulation of risks. It's that simple—and potentially that deadly.

As with heart disease symptoms, what's considered "normal" and "at risk" traditionally has been based on the medical research norm: a 165-pound male. Now, thanks to current research into female-specific heart disease, doctors know that women need their own set of standards. You've heard of these risks, but do you know which ones you gamble with the most?

Smoking Stacks High

We all know that smoking is the most dangerous thing you can do to your heart (and your health in general). But, if you've had a heart attack, it is akin to playing Russian roulette. It is also no surprise that smoking is a hard habit to kick—harder, unfortunately, for women than for men.

Statistics show that 50 percent of all nonfatal heart attacks could be avoided if people would quit smoking. Here is what research says about how the smoking life affects female quality of life:

- ♥ 80 percent of women under the age of 40 who have heart attacks are smokers.

- ♥ Women who are lifetime smokers die an average of 19 years earlier than women who don't smoke.

- ♥ A pack-a-day female smoker under age 44 is seven times more likely to have a heart attack than a woman who never smoked.

- ♥ A pack-a-day female smoker is more than twice as likely to have a heart attack as a pack-a-day male smoker who is the same age.

- ♥ The risk of heart attack is fivefold in women smokers between the ages of 35 and 39.

- ♥ A study of heart attacks in 66,000 women worldwide found that 77 percent were smokers.

- ♥ Smoking reduces levels of heart-protecting estrogen, which can cause early menopause and lower the age at which the risk for heart disease accelerates.

No matter how you cut it, the deck is stacked against female smokers. Smoking is hard on a woman's body. It can cause arteries to constrict, which diminishes the ability of blood to flow. It can raise blood pressure and make the heart beat faster. It lowers levels of good HDL cholesterol and raise levels of bad LDL cholesterol.

Smoking also has other health consequences for women. It is harmful to the reproductive system and increases the chance of hip fractures and osteoporosis later in life. If that isn't enough to give you pause before lighting up, try this: Smoking causes premature wrinkles, dulls hair, makes the skin sallow, and yellows teeth.

Tip 2: **"I Can!" Can Be Your Mantra**

Let's start with the best news first: If you smoke and stop now, you can reverse the damage already done to your heart by half in just one year. In 15 years, it can lower your risk to that of a lifetime non-smoker.

Now, the bad news. For reasons not fully understood, women become more addicted to smoking than men, even though we smoke less, inhale less deeply, and haven't been at it as long (men usually start younger). One theory says it is harder to quit because we find it more satisfying. And we light up for different reasons: to fight stress, ease nervous tension, and keep ourselves from eating—all emotional triggers that make smoking a habit hard to kick.

Just keep on trying. About one-quarter of adult females smoke, which puts us neck-and-neck with men, according to the Centers for Disease Control and Prevention (CDC). If you smoke, most likely you want to quit and have tried many times. Unfortunately, statistics show the success rate for stopping on your own is pretty dismal—less than 10 percent. But there is plenty of help available, from gum, inhalers, and prescription medications to counseling, group therapy, and other professionally run programs. Studies show that among women, combination therapy—a nicotine-withdrawal device (spray, gum, or patch, for instance), prescription drugs, and counseling—increases the likelihood of quitting dramatically.

Tell your daughter this. The CDC reports that smoking has declined 65 percent since the 1960s when the dangers of tobacco first filtered into American consciousness. Great news, if it wasn't for one disturbing fact: Smoking is on the rise among young people,

Playing with Fire

Smoking and birth control pills are a bad combination, but they become life threatening once you turn 35 because they increase your risk of developing blot clots and high blood pressure, and having a stroke.

Though the low-dose pills now available have greatly reduced the overall risk, this is not the case for smokers. Doctors recommend that all women should have a health-risk evaluation before going on the pill and that smokers should consider a different form of birth control.

and it is growing the fastest among teenage girls. Estimates show that 2,000 high-school girls take up smoking every day in the United States. The largest subgroup of smokers is young men and women between the ages of 18 and 24.

Weighing Your Risk

Looked around lately? If you are seeing "more" of people than ever before, it is not an illusion. As a nation, we are fatter than ever, so fat that both the CDC and AHA call it epidemic. Not good, considering obesity is the pied piper of all health problems. But it weighs most heavily on the heart. Statistics show that 77 percent of women who have heart attacks are above normal weight.

Government statistics also show that 61.9 percent of American women are overweight and over half of them—33.4 percent—are considered obese.

Being overweight, and more specifically the things we do to cause it, are associated in some way with everything that is bad for

---

Hip, Hip!

With more than 60 percent of American women overweight, it makes you wonder where all the svelte, thin-hipped women are. New York? Los Angeles? Miami Beach? Any place where models and celebrities roam? Nope.

How about where the buffalo roam. That's right, Colorado. Not only is it the leanest state in the nation, reports the CDC, but also it is the only state in the nation that can boast an average body mass index (BMI) below 25.

the heart. Each thing, in its own way, tears away at the muscle and arteries, causing the heart to age prematurely. Doctors have found aging arteries in obese people as young as 20.

Overweight has been a known villain for decades but the most recent studies show conclusively that the real troublemaker is a specific type of fat—the kind we carry around the middle. It's the apple- rather than the pear-shaped body; the pot-bellied man rather than the bottom-heavy woman. Women generally collect fat in their hips, butts, and thighs. But women can be "apples," too, especially after menopause when their waists tend to thicken.

Tip 3: Waist Away

Are you "safe"? It's easy to find out. Just take a tape measure and wrap it around your naked waist just above the navel. No sucking in the gut! If the number is 35 or above, you're risking trouble.

Be happy to be hippy. Another way to measure your risk is by your waist-to-hip ratio. The cutoff is a ratio of 0.8. If your ratio is below this number, you are in good shape (literally); above it, you have some work to do.

Finding your ratio requires some elementary math: Measure your waist, again just above your navel. Measure your hips at their widest. Divide your waist measurement by your hip measurement. For example:

28-inch waist divided by 38-inch hips = 0.74

Know where you stand. And that is not on your bathroom scale. Scientists have developed a formula using your height and weight measurements to calculate approximate percentage of body fat. It is called the body mass index, or BMI. It does have its flaws, however. For example, it does not differentiate between men and women, and it doesn't take into account frame size—what we call big-boned ver-

BODY-MASS INDEX

Height (ft/in.)	BMI 19–24.9 Normal (lbs)	BMI 25–29.9 Overweight (lbs)	BMI 30 and above Obese (lbs)
5 feet	97–127	128–57	158–79
5'1"	100–131	132–63	164–85
5'2"	104–35	136–68	169–91
5'3"	107–40	141–74	175–97
5'4"	110–44	145–79	180–204
5'5"	114–49	150–185	186–210
5'6"	118–54	155–91	192–216
5'7"	121–58	159–97	198–223
5'8"	125–63	164–202	203–30
5'9"	128–68	169–208	209–36
5'10"	132–73	174–215	216–43
5'11"	136–78	179–221	222–50
6 feet	140–83	184–227	228–58

sus small-boned. But, for now it is the "scale" of choice. So you should know your BMI.

This is not easy to determine unless you happen to be good with numbers. But, take heart. Scientists have figured it out for us. You can find where you stand simply by checking the chart at left

Aim low. Your goal is to be on the lower end of the normal BMI range of 19 to 24.9. Though the risks caused by being overweight develop gradually, a 24 means you are uncomfortably close to where you do not want to be. You don't want to be below 19, either. It's a sign that you may not have enough body fat. (A dream problem, maybe, but one with its own set of health implications.)

Less, but more. It is hard to say which gender is doing better. Overall, there are more overweight men—67.2 percent compared to 61.9 percent of women—but the male obesity rate of 27.5 percent is lower than ours at 33.4 percent.

Be a waist watcher. Recent studies have convinced doctors that abdominal fat is a better indicator of heart disease risk than BMI, so this should be the number you should be concerned about the most. Still, say heart specialists, you should not ignore your BMI. Ideally, you want to be well within the line for both.

Fatal Attraction

Diabetes stalks heart disease, getting more dangerous the closer it gets. And it is on the prowl like never before. The incidence of type 2 diabetes, what used to be known as adult-onset diabetes, has more than doubled since 1994, making it the fastest-growing disease in America.

And women are in the greatest danger.

Science has only recently recognized just how serious this threat is. Data from 450,000 people in 16 countries revealed that women with diabetes are twice as likely to die from heart disease as men with diabetes and they are 2½ times more likely to develop heart disease than women without diabetes. Three-quarters of women with diabetes will end up dying from some form of heart disease.

Type 2 diabetes is characterized by the body's resistance to the normal fluctuations of insulin, a hormone manufactured in the pancreas that helps the body use fuel from food efficiently. Some people are genetically predisposed to diabetes; however, obesity is the major risk factor. Eating large meals and too much sugar cause insulin to work overtime, which taxes the pancreas.

We can't live without insulin. It is secreted during the digestion process to regulate the uptake of glucose into the bloodstream and to orchestrate the efficient use and storage of fat and other nutrients. Resistance, or sensitivity, to insulin disrupts this process and causes, among other things, a cascade of errant glucose to flood the bloodstream. The result can be a host of unpleasant symptoms that cannot be ignored—the most extreme being a stupor that can lead to passing out.

Researchers believe that there is a correlation between the rise in obesity and the rise in the number of people getting type 2 diabetes. So troublesome are the two in combination that doctors have coined a word for them—diabesity.

Tip 4: **Take This Warning Seriously**

Type 2 diabetes is blamed on poor diet, especially one rich in processed sugar and grains. To stop this serious disease before it starts, doctors have introduced a new disease to the medical lexicon: prediabetes. It means your blood sugar level is dancing in the danger zone.

A diagnosis of prediabetes should come as a strong wake-up call. Most people have no idea that they have it until they get their blood glucose checked. It is a warning that if you don't do something to bring your blood sugar down, you most likely will end up with diabetes within 10 years.

Check it out. Make sure that a blood glucose test is part of your yearly blood work-up. Medical guidelines say that the number you want to aim for is below 110mg/dL, but many doctors agree that a better goal is a blood sugar level less than 100mg/dL.

You do not want diabetes. Once it is diagnosed, your life changes dramatically. It means constant supervision of diet and sugar levels and possibly even a need for synthetic insulin. Fortunately, the same kinds of lifestyle changes that are good for the heart also are good for the pancreas.

The Pressure You Don't Need

High blood pressure is an insidious and serious risk factor. It is known as the "silent killer" because it doesn't leave clues as it sneaks up on you. It can be as unpredictable as the stock market—up today, down tomorrow.

When you have high blood pressure, the force of blood against artery walls is stronger than normal. The systolic reading (the top number on your blood pressure reading) measures the pressure of the blood against artery walls when the heart has just finished contracting, or pumping blood. The diastolic reading (the bottom number) is the pressure of your blood against artery walls between beats, when the heart is relaxed and filling with blood.

Ninety percent of the time, doctors aren't even sure what causes

Metabolic Syndrome: The New Risk on the Block

It is also known as metabolic disease or syndrome X, though it is not a disease. Rather, it is a cluster of conditions that together raise the bar on your chances of having a heart attack or dying from heart disease.

You have metabolic syndrome if you are diagnosed with three of the following risks:

- High blood pressure
- Elevated triglycerides
- Excess fat around the waistline
- High cholesterol
- Diabetes
- Prediabetes.

Studies indicate that metabolic syndrome increases with age and is slightly more common among women than men. It is also on the rise among young adults. A population study conducted in Amsterdam showed that by age 36, 10.4 percent of people will have metabolic syndrome.

People with metabolic syndrome have arteries with less flexibility, making it harder for blood to flow. Though medication is available, it is best controlled or avoided through the lifestyle practices suggested in this book.

high blood pressure. But they do know that it wears and tears at the arteries of the heart, setting you up for a heart attack or stroke. According to the AHA, half of the people who have heart attacks and two-thirds of those who have strokes have high blood pressure.

Blood pressure has a tendency to rise with weight gain and is more prevalent in blacks than in whites. It is also widespread. One out of three Americans has it and it is more common in men than women—but only up to a point. At about age 45, the incidence in women gradually increases, and by the age of 60, high blood pressure is more prevalent in women than in men.

It also is more dangerous for women than it is for men because older women are more prone to a stroke. Ideally, your blood pressure should be less than 120/80mmHg. High blood pressure is considered to be greater than 140/90mmHg. Studies, however, show that even a "high normal" reading (systolic between 130 and 139 and diastolic between 80 and 89) can lead to heart problems twice as fast in women than it does in men.

Tip 5: Be Your Own Health Monitor

It usually takes three consecutive high pressure readings in the doctor's office before an official diagnosis is made. Because blood pressure is always fluctuating, you can never be sure that the reading taken in your doctor's office provides an accurate picture of your condition. This makes it difficult for a physician to prescribe the proper medication and the right dosage if you have high blood pressure.

Aim for **blood pressure** no higher than 120/80mmHg.

The solution: You can help your doctor by taking your own blood pressure with an at-home monitor and keeping track of the readings. There are many easy-to-use monitors on the market and you should be able to obtain a reliable one for less than $100. Once you get a monitor, and learn how to use it properly, take your blood pressure every few days for a few weeks, advises Dr. Sheff. Then you can reduce it to about once a week.

Check, check, and check again. If you are concerned that you have high blood pressure or if you are on blood pressure medication, be diligent about checking your pressure about a week before your next doctor's appointment. Write down your readings so you can show your doctor. It will help her diagnose your condition and prescribe medication, if it is needed. Take readings several times each day, making sure to monitor your pressure in the morning, when it is typically at its lowest, and just before bedtime, when it typically starts to drop. Research shows that elevated readings at night are associated with an increased risk of heart disease. The only caveat is that you should not take your blood pressure within an hour after exercise as it will likely be abnormally high for this short interval.

Cholesterol Counting

If lipids (the fat in our blood) were a corporation, women could sue for sexual discrimination. They definitely make us work harder for our payment of good heart health. For example:

- ♥ Women have significantly higher average total cholesterol levels than men, and higher average levels of bad LDL cholesterol.

- ♥ Women need more good HDL cholesterol, the kind that helps get rid of bad LDL, to get the same protection as a man.

- ♥ After menopause, bad cholesterol levels naturally go up and good levels naturally come down.

- ♥ Triglycerides, a type of fat that contributes to high cholesterol, are more harmful in women than in men.

- ♥ Only about one-third of women who should be on cholesterol-lowering drugs are taking them.

A chief cause of high cholesterol is too much fat in the diet, mainly saturated fat. Triglycerides, which are influenced by refined carbohydrates such as sugar, flour, and rice, also adversely affect cholesterol levels. Unfortunately, some women inherit a tendency toward high cholesterol no matter what they eat.

Pregnancy and Cholesterol

A first baby can have a side effect you didn't count on—a drop in good HDL cholesterol. A California study of more than 2,000 women who had given birth for the first time showed an across-the-board drop in HDL that remained in place for up to 10 years. Though more research needs to be done to find out why, researchers believe that changes in hormone levels and fat-cell deposits are involved.

But there is at least some good news: Having additional children does not appear to cause a further drop in HDL.

Cholesterol isn't all bad. It is essential to survival because the body requires it for certain basic functions. For example, it forms a protective sheath around nerve fibers and helps manufacture certain hormones. Because it is essential, the body has the ability to produce all the cholesterol it needs without help from the food chain. So, when we eat fatty foods, we send an extra delivery of cholesterol to the liver where it is processed, turned into fatty acids, and sent out into the bloodstream to go to work. There is some indication that these foods can turn up the natural cholesterol-manufacturing process in the body. This is how we get into cholesterol trouble. The body gets loaded with so much cholesterol that the liver is unable to handle it all. Here is what happens:

Once in the bloodstream, cholesterol teams up with proteins and triglycerides to form a family of fats commonly called lipids. There are two kinds: the hard-working good guys—high-density lipoproteins (HDLs)— and the more sluggish bad guys—low-density lipoproteins (LDLs). Like bank robbers running from the police, LDLs head right for the artery walls where they can hole up 24/7. It takes a posse of HDLs to yank them out and send them back to the liver where they can be expelled from the body. Without enough HDL deputies to corral them, however, the LDLs harden like a gang of criminals with a death wish.

Tip 6: Live the High Life

There is a silver lining in those female arteries. We naturally attract more HDL cholesterol than men. This is significant for several reasons:

- ♥ A high HDL protects us even when total cholesterol is high.

- ♥ A high HDL gives us a lot of years of special protection before HDL naturally heads downward after menopause.

- ♥ It is much harder to increase HDL than decrease dangerous LDL.

It's good to be 50. When it comes to HDL, it's better to be even more than 50mg/dL. Anything below 50 is considered at-risk. For men, risk doesn't start until HDL dips below 45. Consider 50 and above an acceptable challenge. Hint: It's one of the reasons wine and chocolate are good for your heart!

An estimated 50 million women have cholesterol levels considered borderline. That's a lot of cholesterol!

Go as low as you can go. As science learned more about cholesterol through research studies, recommendations for optimal levels of LDL cholesterol started coming down. The current recommendation is to strive to get your LDL as low as it can go. A level of 100 is where risk starts to set in for women. Stay as far from it as possible.

That other fat. When your doctor does a lipids test, she is also testing for triglycerides. For reasons not yet understood, women's hearts are more adversely affected by high triglycerides than men's hearts. For this reason, doctors recommend keeping triglycerides at 100mg/dL or below.

HDL cholesterol should be a minimum of 50mg/dL but the higher, the better. **LDL cholesterol** should not exceed 100mg/dL. The lower, the better.

THE INTERNAL FLAME

> *"Heart disease progresses slowly, and in hindsight, there were a lot of warning signs that I did not recognize."*
> — Jane, age 52

Heart attacks are brought on by plaque buildup in the arteries, which is caused by high cholesterol, which is caused by eating too much saturated fat. Yet, 50 percent of people who have heart attacks have normal cholesterol levels.

Obviously, there are always other risk factors involved—cholesterol is not a lone villain. Still, it is a conundrum that has had scientists searching for clues to another substance that could have it in for our arteries. And they've found one possibility: C-reactive protein (CRP), a molecule that signals low-grade inflammation in the bloodstream.

Inflammation is a natural body response to tissue injury or threats by foreign invaders to healthy cells. For example, any sickness or infection creates inflammation in the body. Chronic conditions such as arthritis can cause it. So, too, can gum disease. By tracking the amount of C-reactive protein in the blood, scientists have found enough evidence to link low-grade inflammation to the process by which fatty deposits attach to and rupture artery walls.

C-reactive protein is manufactured in the liver but scientists at the University of California at Davis Medical Center found that the cells in aortic and coronary arteries also have the ability to produce and secrete it. They found that high levels of the protein can injure cells in the artery walls, which causes plaque to form. High levels of the protein also incite natural inflammation-fighters called cytokines by turning them against healthy cells.

This is a concern because a growing number of studies have found that people with even small elevations of CRP are at risk for heart disease and stroke even in the absence of high cholesterol or other risk factors. Studies also have found that elevated CRP can predict a heart attack in people with unstable angina and those who've had a first attack. Other studies show that high CRP may increase the risk that an artery will close after it has been opened by balloon angioplasty.

Women with high blood pressure are cautioned about inflammation because high CRP puts them at the highest probable risk of having a stroke or heart attack. A study of 14,719 women found that those with metabolic syndrome and high CRP levels are twice as likely to have a heart attack as those who have the syndrome but have low levels of CRP.

The evidence is enough cause for concern that the American Heart Association and the Centers for Disease Control and Prevention now recognize inflammation as a marker to assess heart disease risk.

Tip 7: **Unflame Your Heart**

Detecting inflammation levels can be done through a simple blood test called an hs-CRP, though it is not recommended as a routine screening test. Talk to your doctor about whether or not your CRP should be measured. The results are straightforward:

- ♥ Low risk: A score of 1 or less

- ♥ Moderate risk: A score of 1 to 3

- ♥ High risk: A score above 3

- ♥ A score above 10 means that the cause of the inflammation is unlikely related to heart disease and your doctor should look for an alternative diagnosis such as a recent infection or an autoimmune disease.

DO YOUR GENES FIT?

> "I was 48 years old when I had a heart attack but had only seen gynecologists since I was 18 for all my health care. Not one of them ever mentioned 'heart disease' even though they knew my father and three uncles had died of heart attacks."
> — Elizabeth, age 48

There is no question that heart disease runs in families. Anyone in your immediate family who has had a heart attack makes you a candidate for one. Specifically, risk is considered a concern if your:

- ♥ Father or brother was diagnosed with heart disease before age 55.

- ♥ Mother or sister was diagnosed with heart disease before age 65.

- ♥ Also, there is some evidence that indicates having a mother with heart disease is your bigger concern.

Recent research indicates that there is a familial pattern in the progression of the disease. We can also inherit a predisposition to high blood pressure, high cholesterol, diabetes, stress, weight gain, and certain abnormalities such as how our blood clots. But can we also inherit a tendency to eat poorly and take life a little too easy?

The degree, if any, to which behavior adds to risk is something medical science is still trying to understand. When you think about your family history, also think about your family's habits. Could family habits, and not just family genes, be contributing to the risks you may be taking with your heart?

You can't slip out of your bad genes and pretend they don't belong to you. Heredity is a risk that you should take seriously. If your family genes are against you, it makes it even more important that you create a pro-heart lifestyle. "You can optimize health and prolong life through healthy lifestyle practices, even though you started with a bad genetic load," says patient advocate Dr. Sheff. "For people who are predisposed to cholesterol and high blood pressure, it is critical."

If you don't know your family history, do some investigating. Talk to family members and look at family medical records, if possible. Try to learn about the medical history of your grandparents, parents, aunts, and uncles. The American Heart Association says you should try to find out:

- ♥ History of major medical conditions.

- ♥ Age of onset of major illnesses.

- ♥ Cause and age of death.

- ♥ Ethnic background.

No matter what your current risks are or your family background, making positive changes in the way you live can make a difference. You can start making important changes now. The rest of this book will show you how.

3 Why **Wine** and **Chocolate**

Our mothers, bless them, did everything within their power to make sure we would eat the foods that were good for us. They scolded, they begged, they pleaded, they bribed. "Drink your milk." "Eat your vegetables." Mother was right, of course, but her directives sometimes fell on deaf ears. That's because, too often, it seemed that everything that was good for us had to taste bad.

Nutritional science has come a long, long way in the last couple of generations. Researchers have discovered that food can do a lot more than promote strong and healthy bodies. It can also protect us from a variety of illnesses and even help to reverse the ravages of time and an errant lifestyle. And, yes, food that tastes good can actually be good for us, too. You can now eat to live *and* live to eat.

In the next few chapters, you will learn about a variety of good foods for a healthy heart. You will find out which foods are your heart's guardians and which ones are its rescuers. You will also learn why they do what they do and you will gain important insights into their healing power.

From the long and varied list of heart-healthy foods, let's get right to the two that may have already raised an eyebrow—wine and chocolate. Is it really possible to relax over a drink, satisfy your sweet tooth, and promote a stronger heart at the same time? In a word: Yes!

Here is the message to women from R. Curtis Ellison, M.D., one of America's leading heart researchers: "Americans have long heard that to promote heart health you need to stop eating fat, stop taking in cholesterol, and stop eating things you enjoy. We now have scientific evidence showing that there are many foods you can enjoy and still reduce your risk of heart disease."

Not only are wine and chocolate among them, they are proving to be among the heart's strongest protectors.

WINE: THE NEW HEALTH FOOD

> "After my first heart attack, I gave up butter, white carbo-hydrates, and lost a lot of weight. I quit smoking. After I had my second heart attack, my cardiologist told me to start drinking red wine." —Kathy, age 55

"There is strong scientific evidence that shows moderate drinking promotes heart health," says Dr. Ellison, Chief of Preventive Medicine and Epidemiology and Director of the Institute on Lifestyle and Health at Boston University School of Medicine. "This goes for both women and men, if they've had a heart attack, have heart disease, or want to prevent heart trouble down the road."

Moderate drinking—and this holds true for alcohol in all its consumable forms—promotes a healthy heart in a variety of ways, but its most dramatic effect is its influence on the levels of cholesterol in the blood. "It lowers LDL, the 'bad' cholesterol but, more important, it markedly increases the levels of HDL, the 'good' cholesterol," says Dr. Ellison. Studies show that it can increase HDL by as much as 20 percent.

Studies have also found that moderate drinkers are much less likely to form arterial clots that lead to a heart attack or stroke. And, if clots form, they are more likely to dissolve rapidly in moderate drinkers. Though this has been found true for all alcohol, the most significant benefits come from drinking red wine, says Dr. Ellison.

The Fruit of the Vine

What wine contains and hard liquor lacks are polyphenols, special nutrients found in plant foods. Wine contains more than 500 active substances, but two polyphenols in particular have been the focus of scientific study: resveratrol and saponins. Scientists believe that these substances (and possibly others) work in synergy to alter blood chemistry in ways that help lower cholesterol and prevent other processes that lead to hardening of the arteries. Studies also show that they can help prevent diabetes by reducing sensitivity to insulin, the hormone that controls blood sugar.

The plant of note, of course, is the grape vine. And the wine of choice is red because it is abundantly richer in polyphenols than white. Heart-protecting polyphenols are concentrated in the skin and seeds, which are used in making red wine but are removed to make white wine. Not only do the polyphenols remain, but scientists believe that the fermenting process that turns the grapes into red wine concentrates and expands the action of the nutrients. As a result, the polyphenol content of red wine has been found to be as much as 10 times greater than it is in white.

Tip 8: Drink a Glass of Wine a Day

The operative word in all alcohol consumption is moderation, and for women that means one 5-ounce glass of wine every day or at least 5 days a week, says Dr. Ellison. This is because the beneficial effects may last only 24 to 36 hours after the wine is consumed.

Saving it up so you can drink more once or twice a week just doesn't cut it. "Many people don't drink all week long, then go out on the weekend and binge," says Dr. Ellison. "This is the type of behavior that makes doctors reluctant to recommend drinking as a part of an overall healthy lifestyle."

Go on red. The amount of polyphenols in wine can vary according to the vintage, the type of grape, and where the wine was produced,

---

What's Moderation?

Moderation for women is defined, per day, as:

- 1 glass (5 ounces) of wine, or
- 1 bottle (12 ounces) of beer, or
- 1 cocktail containing 1½ ounces of hard liquor.

For the record, moderation for men is twice these amounts.

---

so it is tough to determine if, say, a cabernet contains more nutrients than a merlot or a pinot noir. Or, for that matter, if California is superior to French or Italian. Perhaps the only given, according to research, is that expensive does not necessarily mean better, at least where polyphenols are concerned. Just select any red wine that you enjoy drinking, says Dr. Ellison.

Some wineries are having their vintages analyzed for resveratrol and saponin content and then advertising their healthfulness. As the public becomes more aware of wine's health advantages you are likely to see certain types being touted for high polyphenol count. At least for now, says Dr. Ellison, including a glass of any type of wine with your evening meal each day is the important thing. If it is a red wine, you get a few extra bonuses from the polyphenols.

Don't stop on white. Many women prefer to drink white wine for its taste and because it complements many foods. "Most white wines have lower levels of the healthy polyphenols that give red wine that additional boost, but they contain approximately the same amount of alcohol, the most important ingredient as far as health effects are concerned," says Dr. Ellison. Wine-makers are already working on ways to improve processing to retain more polyphenols in white wine.

Do as the French do. How can a food-obsessed nation that eats butter, cream, high-fat cheeses, and drinks wine every day also enjoy one of the lowest rates of heart disease in the world? Dr. Ellison, who studied this enigma known as the French Paradox, believes it has a lot to do with the way the French enjoy wine. "The French drink wine as part of their meal," he says. "It is a ritual of the meal. It is part of their lifestyle. And they do it every day."

This is what makes wine the logical drink of choice, he says. "It goes well with food and when you drink along with eating, it cuts down on the adverse effects of alcohol. This is the way it should be."

The French also practice other healthy habits that are good for the heart. They exercise, eat fresh foods, and eat small portions.

Be cordial. If you don't want your daily allotment of wine to disappear too fast, drink it from a small cordial glass. It requires you to take smaller sips and it allows you up to two refills. A cordial glass may not fully reveal the wine's delicate bouquet, but it makes it

When a Good Thing Goes Bad

R. Curtis Ellison, M.D., is the scientist who gained notoriety in 1991 by introducing "the French Paradox" to America on national television. Here's what he knows about drinking, the heart, and longevity:

Moderate drinkers have a lower risk of heart disease and live longer than teetotalers and heavy drinkers. However, there is a point at which a good thing turns into a bad one. In the case of drinking, while people vary in their response to alcohol, women who drink an average of 10 drinks or more a week begin to show adverse effects. "Risk of health problems goes up proportionally with increasing alcohol consumption," Dr. Ellison says.

He also emphasizes that binge drinking has no positive benefits, and can lead to bad behavior and bad health.

easy to savor the drink over a longer period of time.

Not everyone should drink. Although the health benefits of moderate drinking are well-documented, it doesn't mean that teetotalers—those with a drinking problem, certain health problems, or with religious or ethical prohibitions against alcohol—should take it up. Alcohol can also have an adverse effect on women who are overweight, have high blood pressure, or diabetes. As this books shows, there are many other ways for a woman to protect her heart.

Tip 9: Beer Works, Too

An estimated 54 percent of women who drink prefer wine, and though red wine offers the most benefits, similar heart-healthy qualities have been found in beer, says Dr. Ellison. Beer contains alcohol, and the more robust, German-style beers also contain moderate levels of polyphenols.

A group of older women got the opportunity to find out just how good a beer can be. In one study, nine older women and ten middle-age men drank beer every night with dinner for 3 weeks. Protective HDL cholesterol went up an average of 12 percent in both groups—and the women didn't even have to drink as much beer to get the same results as their younger challengers.

The same two groups then drank "near beer," which contains virtually no alcohol, for another 3 weeks. This time, there was no change in HDL levels for either group.

CHOCOLATE IS OUT OF THE BAG

> "I am the poster child for the fact that women are vulnerable to heart disease. I look younger than my age and am very healthy. None of my doctors ever suspected I could have heart disease, even when my cholesterol was over 220."
> —Toni, age 55

Chocolate a healthy food? If you're finding this concept hard to swallow, chew on this: Chocolate has a lot in common with wine when it comes to hidden nutritional treasure. It makes sense, though, when you consider where chocolate comes from—the fruit of a tree.

Chocolate, voted time and again as women's favorite indulgence, comes from the fruit of the cacao tree and contains many of the same heart-saving nutrients found in wine—and then some. No wonder cacao means "food of the gods!"

At least 400 different compounds have been found in chocolate, many of which have long been touted to do a girl good in a variety of specific ways. For example, eating chocolate purportedly releases brain chemicals that can put us in a good mood, mend a broken heart, get us in the mood for love, and massage the wounds of a really bad day. But these are just emotional reasons, or dare we say, excuses to indulge. In recent times, eating chocolate for the heart has taken on a much greater significance.

New scientific data are now evolving showing that chocolate helps fight heart disease. A large number of studies have demonstrated that chocolate, and dark chocolate in particular, can help lower blood pressure, decrease the stickiness of platelets, and improve the function of arteries all of which relate to reducing your risk of getting a heart attack. And preliminary evidence from a study by Dr. Ellison and his colleagues suggests that, whereas nonchocolate candy is associated with an increase in heart disease, higher levels of chocolate intake are associated with up to a 50 percent lower risk of heart disease.

It's the frosting on the chocolate cake, so to speak, that has dared some researchers to suggest that something so decadent can actually bestow health. And here's the real clincher: To get the benefits, you should eat a little every day.

There's just one bitter bite in this near-perfect story. Chocolate is fattening. Just 1 ounce of dark chocolate—the stuff that is best for the heart tops out at about 140 calories, and more than half of those calories come from fat. Talk about the need for moderation!

But let's skip to the good news.

The Bean from the "Forbidden" Tree

Like wine, chocolate is loaded with special nutrients that do the heart good. Specifically, chocolate contains a class of polyphenols called flavanols. This is significant because flavanols are more abundant in dark chocolate than any other food.

Flavanols are concentrated in the cocoa, the solid that is left when the cocoa butter is extracted from cacao beans. The higher the cocoa content, the more bitter the taste. But don't let this put you off. Chocolate connoisseurs will tell you that the cocoa is responsible for the confection's delectable taste.

A study at Pennsylvania State University set out to find just how important cocoa is when it comes to getting heart-healthy benefits. One group of people ate 3½ ounces of dark chocolate a day for 2 weeks, and another group ate the same amount of milk chocolate. Researchers found that polyphenol levels in the blood of the dark chocolate-eaters shot up 20 percent, but it didn't go anywhere in the milk chocolate-munchers.

Similar research in Italy and Scotland found that it takes about twice as much milk chocolate to get the same healthful kick you get from eating dark chocolate. They believe this is because when milk

White is Out

White chocolate isn't chocolate at all. It is missing the ingredient that defines its name: cocoa. And since the health benefits of chocolate are found in the cacao bean, white chocolate contributes nothing to your health.

is added to make the smoother and creamier candy, it binds with the flavanols and prevents them from being absorbed in the bloodstream. In fact, when the same researchers had people drink milk along with dark chocolate, they showed no increase in flavanols in the blood.

This brings us to the big question: How do you eat temptation without going over the limit? The answer: very sensibly.

Tip 10: **Savor the Flavor of Chocolate**

To get health benefits from chocolate, you can eat as little as a half-ounce or an ounce a day, or 2 ounces a few times a week. The amount doesn't matter, says Dr. Ellison, as long as it is dark chocolate and it is eaten within the context of an overall healthy diet—that is, one low in saturated fat and high in vegetables and whole grains.

It should go without saying, but it is being said anyway: Chocolate is not an antidote for a poor diet. In fact, to make chocolate a part of a healthy diet, you should take extra precautions in the other extreme. This takes a two-pronged approach:

One, a day with chocolate means a day you need to be extra vigilant in your choice of other fats. Keep your intake of saturated fats as low as possible. You should balance whatever you're getting in fat and calories from chocolate by cutting back on the fat and calories you would get from eating other foods.

Two, chocolate should not be considered your chief source of flavanols. Leave that up to fruits and vegetables, which we'll discuss later. Rather, eat chocolate, as demonstrated in the studies, to get an extra boost in the number already swimming in your blood.

Go for quality, not quantity. The kind of chocolate used in these scientific experiments is not the kind of chocolate you find near the checkout counter of your local pharmacy. Look for solid dark chocolate—but with no crunchy or creamy centers.

When you think of dark chocolate, what probably comes to mind are the bars you find in the supermarket that are made for cooking. They are classified as bittersweet, semisweet, and sweet and have a high cacao content, which is what you want. However, these bars are not very tasty. There are, however, delicious dark chocolates on the market, and it is one instance where quality does matter.

Go on a health quest. The fun part about the whole healthy chocolate trend is searching for your favorite brand. The one presently scoring major points is Dove Dark, put out by Mars. It is so high in flavanols that it qualifies for use in research studies. Mars uses the logo "Cocoapro" on products that meet its standards for flavanol content. There are many chocolate manufacturers, including Hershey's—the one many of us grew up with—featuring dark chocolate.

As with wine, manufacturers want to take advantage of a good thing, and as chocolate gets more scientific scrutiny, chocolatiers will be hitting the market with new choices.

Long-lasting pleasure. Dark chocolate does not have the melt-in-your-mouth quality of milk chocolate, but that makes it part of the experience. Chop a piece off from a bar (it does not break easily!) and allow it to sit on your tongue for a few moments while it releases its flavors. Take a bite, then let it linger again. You'll sense deeper flavors. You'll even enjoy a lingering taste after you swallow.

To get the most from your chocolate experience, store the candy at a temperature between 60° and 70°F, and eat it at a temperature between 66° and 77°F. Also, eat it when it is fresh.

Wine and chocolate decadently demonstrate that eating for your heart's health can be an interesting and tasty adventure. There are so many delicious foods you can have, there is no reason to even think about what you should not be eating. Chances are, you'll find many you like as much as wine and chocolate.

Dark Chocolate-Covered Strawberries

A dessert that's good for the heart! Chocolate-dipped strawberries are an elegant treat that are deceptively easy to make. One or two will do when a special dinner calls for a special dessert.

3   **ounces semisweet dark chocolate**
1   **teaspoon canola oil**
12 **large, ripe strawberries**

Heat the chocolate in the top of a simmering double boiler until melted, about five minutes. Add the oil and stir until smooth. Dip each strawberry in the chocolate so that it is covered about halfway. Allow any excess chocolate to drip back into the pan.

Layer the strawberries on a platter lined with tinfoil or waxed paper and chill for at least 30 minutes before serving. Make the berries the day you plan to eat them.

4 Eat to Your Heart's Content

Imagine if Mother Earth, with a flick of her wand, could render all the land's edibles into heart-healthy, mouth-pleasing morsels. What would it mean to women's health?

Quite a lot, it seems. It would reduce female heart disease by more than three-quarters and add nearly 5 years to our lives.

And guess what? No magic wand is required. All we need to do is eat richly from Mother Earth's vast heart-saving food supply as part of an overall healthy diet. It's proof-positive of the heart-protecting power of food.

Many of the world's heart problems possibly could be erased, or at least delayed, by eating certain foods, according to a team of researchers from various parts of the world who wanted to find out what effect a heart-smart diet would have on the rate of heart disease. The scientists first designed a hypothetical, modern, heart-healthy menu of seven foods. Then, they went back to 1948 and the beginning of the now well-known Framingham (Massachusetts) Heart Study that followed the lifestyle habits and the progression of cardiovascular disease among 5,209 residents, including 2,873 women. Using what they called a life table, they recoded the Framingham data to measure the potential impact their hypothetical diet would have on the world today.

The result: A drop of 76 percent in heart disease for both men and women. They also found women could enjoy an additional 8.1 years of heart disease-free living and actually increase their overall lifespan by 4.8 years. The foods used in the study, which they coined the Polymeal, were red wine, dark chocolate, fish, fruits, vegetables, garlic, and almonds.

"We selected these foods because they each possess a substance that benefits the heart in a special way," said lead researcher, Oscar H. Franco, M.D., of the University Medical Center Rotterdam in the Netherlands. "We believe any of the foods known to have a heart-health effect would have similar results. The bottom line is that

Men Have the Edge

Women fared well but men actually fared better on the experimental heart-healthy Polymeal, according to research results.

	Women	Men
Increase in Life Expectancy	4.8 years	6.6 years
Increase in Life Free of Heart Disease	8.1 years	9 years
Decrease in Life Expectancy as a Result of Heart Disease	3.3 years	2.4 years

these foods, or any heart-healthy foods, as part of an otherwise low-fat healthy diet, can have a major impact on the prevention of heart disease."

Dr. Franco and his associates also proved that each food independently makes its own contribution to heart health. They demonstrated this when they set out to see what would happen if they removed just one of the seven foods from the diet. For each food taken away, the rate of heart disease crept back up. It showed that some were more effective than others—notably wine and chocolate.

The appealing thing about the Polymeal is that the foods on it are, well, so appealing. They are also foods enjoyed by some of the world's healthiest cultures. Fish, fruits, wine, almonds—not bad for starters. But wait until you see what else is on the menu!

THE MEDITERRANEAN STYLE

> "I am the only diabetic in my family and, like many people with diabetes, I'd heard all the warnings about my kidneys, my eyes, and my limbs. No one mentioned the most dangerous risk of diabetes: heart disease." — Maria, who had a heart attack at age 44

The ancient town of Palekastro is nestled among miles of olive groves between the mountains and deep blue sea on the sunny isle of Crete, just south of Greece. While other towns have made room for large resorts and tourist traffic, the people of tiny Palekastro have managed to keep their old-fashioned ways, including the daily ritual of gathering in one of the town's many tavernas to enjoy food, drink,

The Power of Food

The seven foods that comprised the Polymeal individually contributed a potential reduction in the risk of heart disease:

Food	Amount per Day	Reduced Risk
Red wine	5 oz.	32%
Garlic	1-2 cloves	25%
Chocolate	3½ oz.	21%
Fruits & vegetables	14 oz.	21%
Fish	4 oz. (4 times a week)	14%
Almonds	2½ oz.	12.5%

and companionship after a hard day's work.

As a result of their lifestyle, Cretian life expectancy is among the highest and their heart-disease rate among the lowest in the world. It's no wonder, then, that the people of Crete and the surrounding European nations have been fascinating heart researchers since World War II. They are now considered role models of exemplary eating habits.

One study of 22,000 Greeks showed that those who adhered most closely to the traditional Mediterranean diet had the lowest risk of heart disease. Most recently a study of 74,000 aging Mediterraneans found that those truest to the traditional diet can expect to live longer than their contemporaries who have adopted different eating habits.

The traditional Greek diet is pretty much limited to what can be acquired locally—fish and seafood, fruits, vegetables, breads created from whole grains, legumes, nuts, and seeds. Meat, if eaten at all, is used for flavor rather than as the star of the meal. Greeks generally drink wine moderately and always as part of a meal. Their dessert, when served, is simply fruit. And, of course, there is the ubiquitous and flavorful olive. It is the olive, or more precisely its oil, that researchers believe plays a leading role in their long lives and strong hearts.

The Mighty Monos

Greeks are known to pour olive oil as freely as the French pour wine, meaning that the Greek diet, in spite of all its good fruits and vegetables, is not exactly low fat. This led researchers to the conclusion that it is the type of fat, rather than the amount of fat, that draws the line between good and bad.

Fat comes in three varieties: saturated, polyunsaturated, and monounsaturated. We have long been taught that the saturated fat in meats, butter, and other animal-based foods is a major contributor to the plaque that clogs our arteries. Olive oil, on the other hand, is brimming with monounsaturated fat. And therein lies the difference. Monos are heart healthy. They help reduce the amount of bad LDL cholesterol swimming in your arteries and, more important, help to fortify good HDL cholesterol. Some studies show that monos can even raise HDL.

In one Spanish study, women followed three different high-fat diets for a month at a time. For the first month, they used butter, high in saturated fat; the second month they used olive oil, high in monounsaturated fat; and the third month they used sunflower oil, high in polyunsaturated fat. Cholesterol went up on the butter

Include 1 to 3 tablespoons of **olive oil** a day in your diet.

diet—no surprise there. The women's total and LDL cholesterol fell on both the olive oil and sunflower oil diets, but protective HDL cholesterol went up only on the mono diet.

Tip 11: Pour On the Olive Oil

Consider it a lube job for the heart. The body needs a certain amount of fat, so give it only the best. You wouldn't expect a Ferrari to run on diesel fuel, would you?

A healthy dose. At 120 calories per tablespoon, olive oil is an expensive way to spend your calories. But, it is also full-flavored, and a little can go a long way. So what's enough? Nutritionists and heart experts differ on what should be an optimum daily dose, but Olga Raz, R.D., a registered dietitian who has done nutritional research on women's heart health in Israel, believes it should be between 1 and 3 tablespoons a day. "It's a lot, I know, but olive oil is important," she says.

Go for quality. The quality of olive oil is based on its acid content. As acid content goes up, quality comes down. Most of the world's olive oil is produced in the southern regions of Greece, France, Spain,

The Test for Purity

To make sure the quality of your olive oil is what it says it is, put a small amount of oil in a glass and put it in the refrigerator for 24 hours. If the oil becomes gel-like, then it is mostly olive oil. It the sample remains liquid, there are other oils in the bottle. It is not pure olive oil.

All Heart Vinaigrette

Classic vinaigrette does not contain garlic or citrus, but adding them makes it all the better for the heart.

- 1 **clove garlic, minced**
- 1 **teaspoon Dijon mustard**
- ¼ **cup red wine vinegar**
- ¾ **cup extra-virgin oil olive**
- ½ **teaspoon fresh thyme**
- ½ **teaspoon lemon juice**

Mix the garlic, mustard, and vinegar in a small bowl. Using a whisk, slowly add the oil. Stir in the thyme and lemon juice. Pour into a glass cruet with a tight-fitting lid and refrigerate. Bring to room temperature and shake well before using.

and Italy. But it's also made in California. Connoisseurs say small family-run operations turn out the finest oils because they are most likely to follow old-time manufacturing customs.

The best olive oils come from the first pressing and range from golden yellow to almost bright green in color. The greener the oil, the less acid it contains.

Extra-virgin olive oil has the least acid at 1 percent. Virgin olive oil has an acid level no greater than 3 percent. It has a low smoke point, so be careful when using it in the sauté pan. Don't let the heat get too high.

Pure olive oil is the lowest of the breed and comes from the second or third pressing. It has an acidity content no higher than 4 per-

Ranking the Fats

Olive oil should be your fat of choice because it has no match when it comes to monounsaturated fat. Monos have been found to help lower LDL cholesterol and raise heart-healthy HDL cholesterol. Polyunsaturates are healthy as well and can help reduce total cholesterol. They appear to have little or no value in increasing HDL. Saturated fats are fat felons, charged with supplying substances that cling to and clog up arteries. Oils, however, contain no cholesterol. Butter, on the other hand, is not only high in saturated fat, but it is also high in cholesterol at 31.5 milligrams per tablespoon.

Here are how the fats measure up, based on grams per tablespoon. For the record, oils contain approximately 120 calories per tablespoon and butter 102 calories.

Fat	Mono-unsaturated	Poly-unsaturated	Saturated
Almond oil	9.5	2.4	1.1
Avocado oil	9.9	1.9	1.6
Butter	3.3	0.4	7.2
Canola oil	8.3	4.1	1.0
Coconut oil	0.8	0.2	11.8
Corn oil	3.3	7.9	1.7
Cottonseed oil	2.4	7.0	3.5
Olive oil	10.0	1.2	1.9
Palm oil	5.0	1.3	6.7
Peanut oil	6.2	4.3	2.3
Safflower oil	1.7	10.1	1.2
Sesame oil	5.4	5.7	0.9
Sunflower oil	2.7	8.9	1.4

cent and a high smoke point—410°F—so it is the best for cooking.

What the French say. Extra-virgin, nonfiltered olive oil is purported to be the healthiest of all. It appears cloudy and slightly thick, and the label bears the words *huile d'olive vierge extra nonfiltre*. It is also the most expensive. Extra-virgin has a low smoke point—250°F. It is also expensive, so save it for dishes in which you can really appreciate the flavor, such as for salad dressings, in sauces, and as a flavoring on steamed or grilled vegetables.

Keep it cool. Monounsaturated fats have a chemical structure that makes them delicate by nature. It means that olive oil can turn rancid easily. Don't buy it in large bottles if you don't plan to use it daily. You can extend the life of your olive oil by storing it in a cool, dark place. Also, keep the oil in a dark bottle because light is as bad for it as the heat.

Tip 12: One Olive, Hold the Gin

Auntie Mame of theater fame shunned olives because they took up too much room in her martini glass. She didn't know what she was missing. Olives take a rap because of their high fat content but we now know that monos make a big fat difference. Ten olives are a whole lot better than 10 potato chips which, piece for piece, have more calories and lots of unhealthy fat.

Eating the fruit also gives you the benefit of any phytochemicals it contains. Phytochemicals, special nutrients present in sun-soaked plants, act as antioxidants by helping to slow down the buildup of plaque on artery walls. The downside is that olives contain a lot of salt, so they should not be part of a low-sodium diet. Here are some ways to spread the goodness and spread out the calories and salt.

- ♥ Toss olives in salads and pasta or slice them and put them on sandwiches.

- ♥ Add olives to stir-fries. They go particularly well with chicken.

- ♥ Mix olives in risottos and rice pilafs.

- ♥ For a special treat, combine several varieties of olives with a few slices of lemon zest and a fresh sprig of rosemary and warm them in pure olive oil for a cocktail-hour snack.

Tip 13: **Make Room for Canola, Too**

Canola oil is arguably as good as olive oil in terms of heart health; it just doesn't get as much good press. Canola is not as high in monounsaturated fat as olive oil, but it has more than three times the polyunsaturated fat and nearly half as much saturated fat. Studies show that it is as effective as olive oil in lowering total and bad LDL cholesterol without affecting good HDL cholesterol.

Canola is also more user-friendly. It is much cheaper than olive oil; its flavor is milder; and it will not wither under high heat. As with olive oil, it should be kept in a cool place.

Tip 14: **Add Nuts to the Mix**

Dr. Franco did not put olive oil on his Polymeal menu, but he could have. Instead almonds were his monounsaturate of choice. Almonds are also part of the Mediterranean diet and get a lot of credit for contributing to the low rate of heart disease. Studies show that they also have the ability to lower total and bad LDL cholesterol.

Several studies with both almonds and walnuts have proven again that a diet can be high in fat as long as the fat is monounsaturated. Researchers put a group of men and women on a low-fat, low-cholesterol diet, featuring lots of fruits and vegetables, for 2 weeks. Then, they upped their fat intake by adding 3 ounces of raw almonds to their daily diet. This meant they were getting 37 percent of their calories from fat. After 3 weeks on the high-fat diet, their total cholesterol and LDL cholesterol levels came down. The protective HDL cholesterol was not affected at all. A study in Spain produced similar results with walnuts.

In fact, almost any nut will have a similar beneficial effect. The Nurses' Health Study, which has followed the dietary habits of 121,600 nurses between the ages of 30 and 55 since 1976, found that women who ate nuts on almost a daily basis had half the heart attack risk of nurses who rarely ate them.

A healthy dose. Studies suggest that eating a handful of nuts—about 1 ounce—five times a week lowers the risk of heart attack by 50 percent. And monos are not the only good reason to eat them. Almonds are high in fiber and are a rare source of vitamin E, and plant sterols, both heart-healthy food substances. They are also an excellent vegetarian source of protein.

Mix them up. Walnuts, pecans, almonds, macadamia—any kind of nuts are good sources of monos. Just make sure you eat them plain. Nuts are a high-calorie food, so eating honey-roasted and other flavor-enhanced varieties defeats their healthful purpose. Sprinkle nuts on salads, add them to stir-fries, and put them in your cereal and yogurt.

Tip 15: Go Easy on Poly

Polyunsaturated oils are sort of half-good and half-bad. They are good because they help reduce dangerous LDL cholesterol but not so good because they can bring down protective HDL cholesterol as well. Safflower, sunflower, and corn oils are three of these "in-between" oils.

The reason these oils act so strangely is because they contain phytosterols, natural chemicals that are similar in composition to cholesterol. As a result, the body mistakes sterols for cholesterol and tries to absorb them. Only it doesn't happen. That's good because it also means the body can't absorb the cholesterol, either.

The bad news is that sterols can block absorption of the good cholesterol in addition to the bad, so use these oils sparingly.

The Black List
The following are words associated with the fats you should avoid:

- Butter
- Coconut oil
- Hydrogenated
- Lard
- Margarine
- Palm oil
- Saturated
- Shortening
- Tropical oils

Tip 16: **Use the Better Bread Spread**

You know to stay away from butter and margarine. But an artificial butter-like spread came out not too long ago that is actually good for you because it can help lower cholesterol. It has the same texture and tastes similar to regular tub margarines, but it is made using chemically modified sterols. Two brand names are Benecol and Take Control. About 2 tablespoons a day have been found to help reduce cholesterol by 10 percent. But they are not cheap. An 8-ounce container, or 16 one-tablespoon servings, costs around $5. (Plant sterols are also available in gel caps as a supplement.)

A Rose for the Heart

It's unfortunate that garlic is called the "stinking rose" because of its pungent odor. It deserves better because this herb is true-blue when it comes to doing favors for the heart.

In the Polymeal, a clove or two a day had the ability to bring down heart disease by up to 25 percent. Here's why it is so special.

Tip 17: **Have a Heart for Allicin**

When you smash a clove of garlic, you are releasing allicin, a compound with many benefits, including the ability to fight bacteria and viruses and protect the heart.

Eating garlic regularly has been shown to help reduce heart-attack risk by lowering bad LDL cholesterol and triglycerides in the blood without affecting good HDL. It also can reduce the risk of stroke by helping to break up substances that cause clots.

Add garlic to your diet; ideally at least a clove a day.

A healthy dose. Studies show that eating a clove or more per day as part of a healthy diet can help reduce total cholesterol from 10 to 25 percent. A study in Kuwait found that eating three cloves a day can decrease the risk of heart disease by 20 percent.

Crush, chop, or mince. Any way you use garlic is fine. As long as you can smell it, you know you are getting the benefit.

Fresh is best. Studies show that dried garlic, garlic powder, and garlic salt are not nearly as effective as fresh garlic and possibly may offer no benefit at all. On the other hand, garlic capsules, which emit no odor, have been found to have a benefit similar to eating fresh garlic.

Enjoy real garlic bread. If you can't imagine biting into a whole clove of garlic, you haven't tried roasted garlic. Roasting reduces the taste from strong to mellow and makes it easy to spread on whole-grain bread. You get great tasting garlic bread without the butter.

A SEA OF HEALTH

"I am a 42-year-old African American. I had a heart attack in my late twenties but it wasn't diagnosed until I was 38."
— Marguerite

For centuries, as southern Europeans fished heart-healthy sustenance from the warm Aegean and Mediterranean seas, the Eskimos in Greenland were poking holes in the Arctic ice looking for their

Roasted Garlic

You'll be amazed by the mild taste when garlic is made this way. And it won't leave a lingering odor reminiscent of an Italian restaurant.

- **1 large head garlic**
- **1 tablespoon olive oil**

Preheat the oven to 350°F.

Cut the top off the head of garlic to expose the cloves. Remove any flaky skins but make sure most of the skin remains intact.

Pour the oil in a dish and swirl the garlic head around to cover it completely in oil.

Wrap the garlic head tightly in aluminum foil, put it on a baking sheet and bake for 50 minutes to 1 hour. It will feel soft when it is finished.

Open the foil and let the garlic cool for a few minutes before handling.

Now this is the fun part. Pull off a clove or two and pop it out of the skin and spread it onto a piece of dark bread. It makes a great snack.

own food. The Eskimos didn't have sun-kissed land to farm, so they pretty much had to depend on the bounty from the icy sea.

Even fish need insulation in Arctic water, so the ones with the best survival rates were those with fat in their tissues. Fatty fish became the mainstay of the Eskimo diet and, in turn, added fat to the Eskimos. This eventually attracted the attention of heart researchers because they noticed that Eskimos had a lower-than-expected rate of heart disease, even though they dined regularly on fatty fish, including whale blubber.

Calling on the Omegas

The researchers discovered that cold-water fish contain special substances, called omega-3 fatty acids, which serve as a kind of antifreeze that protects fish in the cold water. They also found that it is just as special to the human heart. Omega-3s accumulate in cell membranes where they keep watch over the rhythmic ticking of the heart. They help to normalize heart rate when an outside influence tries to rev it up or make it skip a beat.

Omega-3s work so well they can even help slow the racing heartbeat that causes life-threatening ventricular fibrillation. While in residence, omega-3s keep blood clots at bay, and there is evidence that they also help slow the growth of plaque in arteries, lower triglyceride levels, improve blood pressure, and strengthen blood vessels. They may even be helpful in preventing sudden death from heart attack.

Not only are cold-water fish a rich source of omega-3s, they are the only source of the most important two, eicosapentaenoic acid (EPA) and docosahexaenoic acid (DHA). There is no recommended daily intake for omega-3s but nutrition experts say 1,000 milligrams a day is a protective amount.

Eat fish rich in omega-3 fatty acids 3 to 5 times a week.

King Fish

The leading sources of omega-3 fatty acids per 4-ounce serving:

- ♥ Herring   2,347 mg.
- ♥ Sardines   1,786 mg.
- ♥ Salmon   1,473 mg.
- ♥ Mackerel   1,273 mg.

- ♥ Trout   1,213 mg.
- ♥ Halibut   933 mg.
- ♥ Tuna   785 mg.

Tip 18: **Treat Yourself to Fish**

The many benefits of fish could be ours if only we ate more of it. People who keep tabs on such things say that Americans eat fish on an average of only once every 10 days. That's not very good when you consider that the 84,068 admitted fish lovers in the Nurses' Health Study—those who reported eating fish five or more times a week— had a heart attack risk 34 percent lower than nurses who ate fish less than once a month.

A healthy dose. Polymeal researchers found that eating 4 ounces of fish four times a week can help reduce heart disease by 14 percent. The American Heart Association (AHA) recommends that those with heart disease eat fish three to five times a week. To help protect a healthy heart, the AHA recommends fish at least twice a week.

To get the maximum benefits of EPA and DHA found in fish:

Savor salmon. Salmon isn't the best source of omega-3s, but it is the most popular. Americans by far are the biggest salmon-eaters. According to the Institute for Health and the Environment, we eat 207,000 metric tons a year. A 4-ounce serving of salmon contains 1,473 milligrams of omega-3s.

Farmed a toxic shock? The increase in commercial fish farming has raised two health concerns. Studies have found that farmed salmon contain more environmental toxins than those caught in

Bill's Baked Salmon with Spinach and Herbs

My friend Bill Price loves salmon but he never makes it the same way twice. He lets what is fresh from the garden dictate how he'll develop the recipe. Fresh wild salmon is so succulent, he says to never disguise it with a sauce. The idea is to keep it simple. You can substitute any of these ingredients with whatever you have fresh in the garden.

1	bunch fresh spinach leaves, washed and dried
1½	pounds skinless wild salmon fillet
2	tablespoons low-fat mayonnaise
3	tablespoons extra-virgin olive oil
4	sprigs fresh marjoram
4	sprigs fresh rosemary
½	cup snipped fresh chives

Preheat a grill or the oven to 400°F.

Lay out a piece of heavy-duty aluminum foil large enough to hold the salmon. Spread the spinach down the center of the foil so it is the same length as the salmon. Place the salmon on top of the spinach. Spread a thin layer of mayonnaise on top of the fish. Drizzle with the oil. Scatter the marjoram, rosemary, and chives on top. Bring the foil ends up lengthwise and secure all the edges, tent-style. Place on a hot grill or in the oven for about 20 minutes.

Serves 4 to 6.

the sea because the close breeding grounds are more attractive to contaminants. They also lack the buttery-textured flesh of wild salmon, a sign that they contain less omegas-3s. Supermarkets are the most popular outlet for farm-raised salmon, according to the Institute for Health and the Environment.

Go wild. Wild salmon is fins and tails superior to farm-raised salmon. It has more flavor and also contains the most omega-3s. It is also the most expensive, sometimes running as much as $20 a pound.

Check their passport. Unfortunately, recent reports claim that farmed salmon is often passed off as wild. If in doubt, ask your fishmonger where the salmon was fished. If it's from Chile, it is most likely farmed. Chile is the world's second-largest producer of farm-raised salmon, and most of the salmon sold in the United States comes from Chile or Canada.

Dine out on it. The best and freshest fish are often put aside for restaurants whose customers are willing to pay the high price. A survey of fine-dining establishments in the United States shows that 70 percent put salmon on the menu. Ask if the salmon is wild before ordering.

And the runners-up are . . . To outdo salmon in omega-3 content, you'd have to eat the same amount of herring or sardines. That's a lot of sardines!

Fish and the PCB Factor

Does it really make sense for women to eat a lot of fish, considering the findings that many fish are polluted with methylmercury and polychlorinated biphenyls (PCBs)?

Current thinking is that the heart-healthy benefits of eating fish far outweigh the risks, with two exceptions: Pregnant women and those who are nursing. The Food and Drug Administration and Mayo Clinic recommend that these women avoid eating large fish because they contain greater concentrations of the poisons in their fat cells. Large fish include king mackerel, shark, swordfish, tilefish, and fresh tuna. On the other hand, it's okay to eat shrimp, salmon, pollock, and catfish, but not more than a total of 12 ounces a week. These species are known to have low levels of PCBs.

As for canned tuna, albacore (white) is higher in mercury than light tuna. If you simply must have albacore, Mayo Clinic suggests limiting it to 6 ounces a week.

Tip 19: **Hold the Fish-and-Chips**

If you want the healthy benefits of fish, forget frying. In one study, researchers compared the omega-3 fatty acid levels in people who routinely ate fish baked or broiled and those who ate fish fried. Blood levels of omega-3s were significantly higher in the fish-eaters who preferred it baked or broiled than in those who preferred it fried. The researchers believe that frying reduces the omega-3 content of the fish.

EARTHLY PLEASURES

"After a routine blood test, my doctor called and asked me to come over to her office immediately because my cholesterol reading was 330. I had no idea why she was so upset."
— Ellen, age 55

It was an experiment that lasted only four weeks and included just 46 people, but the results indicate that certain foods can be basically as effective as a drug when it comes to controlling dangerously high cholesterol.

The study, conducted at the University of Toronto, divided the people—all with high cholesterol—into three groups, each with a special diet. One group was put on a standard cholesterol-lowering diet consisting of low-fat foods and whole-wheat grains. The second group ate the same diet but also took the cholesterol-lowering drug, lovastatin. The third group followed an experimental vegetarian diet developed by the researchers that featured soy foods in place of meat and a special type of fiber found in oats and barley. They called it the Portfolio Diet.

After 4 weeks, people on the standard diet had an 8 percent reduction in bad LDL cholesterol and a 10 percent drop in C-reactive protein, a marker for subclinical chronic inflammation, which is now believed to be a predictor of heart disease. The people on the standard diet and cholesterol medication had a 30.9 percent drop in LDL and a 33.3 percent reduction in C-reactive protein. The Portfolio dieters reduced LDL by 28.6 percent and C-reactive protein by 28.2 percent.

These results are significant, noted lead researcher Dr. David J. A. Jenkins, because it shows that certain foods eaten in the right combination can get nearly the same results as certain cholesterol-lowering medications. The foods that did the job?

- ♥ Oat bran and other oat products

- ♥ Legumes, such as beans

- ♥ Soy food products, such as soy burgers, in place of meat

- ♥ Soy milk instead of cow's milk

- ♥ Psyllium (a special kind of fiber)

- ♥ Sterol-containing butter substitutes Benecol and Take Control

- ♥ Almonds

- ♥ Walnuts

- ♥ Fruits

- ♥ Vegetables

All the foods contain special compounds that have the strength on their own to fight cholesterol. As a group, however, they have the power to knock it down.

Fiber Power

Fiber is the part of the plant food the body can't digest. It passes through the system pretty much intact. There are two types of fiber: soluble and insoluble. All plant foods contain both, although wheat grains have more insoluble fiber and oat grains are most abundant in soluble fiber. This is an important difference because studies have found that soluble fiber plays a special role in fighting cholesterol.

Tip 20: **Feel Your Oats**

Notice how oatmeal gets sticky when you add water or milk? That's soluble fiber in action. In spite of its name, soluble fiber does not dissolve in liquid, but when it gets into a liquid environment, it absorbs liquids from the foods you eat and from the gastrointestinal tract. Don't forget, the body is 60 percent water and the digestive system contains a lot of it. So the fiber absorbs the liquid readily on the trip through the gut, through the colon, and out of the body. That collection basket includes cholesterol. Here's why:

As mentioned in chapter 2, the body requires a certain amount of cholesterol. This is because the liver uses it to make bile acids to help the digestion process. When soluble fiber meets up with bile

If you have high cholesterol, get 10 to 25 grams of **soluble fiber** a day.

acids, it binds with them and takes them along for the ride out of the body. As a result, the liver must call in more cholesterol to make more bile acids, thereby reducing the amount of cholesterol in your system. In addition to oats, soluble fiber is found in beans, peas, barley, fruit, and flaxseed.

A healthy dose. Health organizations and research experts recommend that we get 25 grams a day of dietary fiber, though they don't specify which kind. If you have high cholesterol, however, doctors recommend that you concentrate your effort on soluble fiber.

Studies suggest that eating just 10 grams of soluble fiber a day can reduce cholesterol by up to 5 percent.

Eat your oatmeal. Half the fiber in oat bran is soluble, so it is your best source of this cholesterol-buster. In addition, eating oatmeal is just a great healthy way to start the day, because it is so darn healthy (if you don't add butter or sugar). Quaker has instant oatmeal that offers 4 to 5 grams of soluble fiber per serving.

Add a little fruit. Most fruit contains both soluble and insoluble fiber, so you can up your breakfast portion of fiber by adding fresh fruit. Raisins, blackberries, blueberries, and apples contain soluble fiber and go well with oatmeal.

Your daily bread. If you don't like oatmeal, try oat meals. Buy oat bran bread or make oatmeal muffins and cookies. The key here is to make your own. Unless you know for certain that store-bought oat products don't contain any saturated fats or trans fats, you can end up canceling out your good intentions.

Tip 21: Pick a Peck of Pectin

You might be familiar with pectin as the goo that puts the gel in jelly. Pectin is a type of soluble fiber that gives apples the reputation for keeping the doctor away. Pectin does the same good things for the heart that oats do. Adding fruit to your diet is a great way to increase your fiber intake.

An apple a day... will help keep heart disease at bay. In one study, 30 men and women in France ate two to three apples a day for a month. Their total cholesterol dropped an average of 14 percent. One medium apple contains nearly 2 grams of pectin. In addition to being rich in pectin, apples also contain another cholesterol-buster called flavanoids, a large group of nutrients with antioxidant properties.

Pear away. If you get tired of apples, or don't particularly like them, eat pears. Bite for bite, they contain almost as much pectin and flavanoids as apples.

Tip 22: Beans, Beans at Any Meal

If there's a food that gets no respect, it's the bean. For centuries it was considered the fare for peasants and paupers who could not afford the meat and game enjoyed by the upper class. But those beans get at least some of the credit for cultivating the "hardy peasant stock" that generations since have been lucky to inherit, for the lowly, inexpensive bean is almost priceless when it comes to the heart.

Beans deserve a special status as a healthy food because they are a rich source of cholesterol-clobbering soluble fiber and a rare vegetable protein. Studies have found that eating beans regularly in your diet can bring down total cholesterol and triglyceride levels with no harmful effect on protective HDL cholesterol levels.

No one wants to live by beans alone, but Mother Earth gave us enough varieties to make it possible!

Beans every way. There are adzuki and alfalfa, broad and black, lentils and limas, chickpeas and split peas, navy and Great Northern. And that's just for starters. The truth is, if you had to eat beans every day, you really could. The varieties in which you can get 2 grams or more in a ½-cup serving include black beans, cranberry beans, kidney beans, lima beans, navy beans, and lentils.

Canned is okay. This is a convenience and shortcut you don't want to ignore. Give them a rinse, though, as they tend to contain a lot of sodium.

Veto Mexicano. Refried beans are on heart disease's most-wanted list. That's because otherwise perfectly good pinto beans are mashed and not just fried, but fried in lard! There are canned vegetarian and nonfat refried beans on the market, however, that are reportedly quite tasty. So, if you love refried beans and can't do without them, give these a try.

If you love Mexican treats, you can still make heart-healthy points by ordering a burrito with beans (not refried) instead of beef.

The cassoulet caste. Leave it to the French to elevate the humble bean to gourmet status. Named for the earthenware vessel in which it is made, cassoulet is a composite of a variety of meats slow-cooked in a base of white beans (and, unfortunately, sometimes goose fat). French culinary lore claims that pots of cassoulet could live on the stove for years as a day's subtraction would be replaced with fresh additions. Lore also claims that every family throughout the Languedoc, where the dish originated, has its own version and no two are alike! It is a perfect example of the vast possibilities for bean cuisine.

Cassoulet as the French enjoy it is not what you'd consider

Chili con Kathy

After my friend Kathy Herbein had a heart attack at age 54
she redesigned the way she ate and cooked. She did it so
cleverly that no one noticed she had trimmed the fat in the
family's favorite recipes. She keeps this heart-healthy version
of spicy turkey chili in her refrigerator at all times. It makes a
quick lunch and is always there when she needs a few bites
of something throughout the day. She has redesigned chili
into an effortless task.

- 1 **Vidalia onion, chopped**
- 1 **tablespoon olive oil**
- 2 **cloves garlic, minced**
- 1 **pound ground turkey breast**
- 3 **15.5 ounce cans pink, red, or black
     kidney beans, rinsed**
- 2 **8-ounces cans chopped tomatoes, with juice**
- 1 **teaspoon chili powder**
- ¼ **teaspoon cumin**
- ¼ **teaspoon Tabasco sauce (optional)**
- ½ **cup chopped fresh cilantro or parsley**

In a heavy-bottomed casserole, sauté the onion in the oil
until soft, about 5 minutes. Add the garlic and cook 1 minute.
Add the turkey and continue cooking, until the meat is just
cooked through. Add the beans, tomatoes (with juice), chili
powder, cumin, and Tabasco, if using. Lower the heat, cover,
and cook for 30 to 40 minutes. Add the cilantro or parsley.

Serves 8.

health food, but it can be. And it is a fun dish to make. Try making a heart-healthy version by replacing the fat with olive oil. Replace the fatty, heavy meats with lean pork and skinless chicken thighs, and the pork sausage with fresh turkey sausage. Add extra beans or try the vegetarian version recommended on page 98.

Tip 23: Spice It Up at Home

You can't get more down-home than chili, so why not turn this family favorite into a heart-pleaser with just a few adjustments. Substitute turkey or chicken for the beef and add extra beans.

Just make sure that you spice it up. Chili is great for the heart because of its namesake—chili peppers. Capsaicin, the substance that gives chiles their spicy kick, has been found to have a whole lot of health benefits, including helping to reduce triglycerides. A low-fat chili recipe can be found on page 93.

Tip 24: Get Your Wheat as Well

Beans, apples, oats. Sounds like a pretty tasty way to store up on fiber, doesn't it? Sad to say, it isn't happening. We don't do a good job of getting any kind of fiber, insoluble or soluble, on a daily basis. The average woman eats only 13.6 grams of fiber a day (men get 17.8 grams). The reason? We are selecting refined flour over fiber-filled flour.

Lack of dietary fiber was not an issue until after the Civil War, when the steel roller made the refining of flour a cheap and easy process. Refinery mills started turning out soft white flour, a stark contrast to the brown, gritty flour people were accustomed to working into their daily breads and porridges. White flour was considered a revolutionary invention until the second half of the 20th century, when scientists realized what it was doing to sound nutrition.

When grains are processed, two of the three layers—the bran and the germ—are removed, taking the fiber and nutrients with them. That leaves only the starch layer, which is known as the endosperm. Manufacturers have solved the nutrition issue by fortifying cereals with plenty of vitamins and minerals. But they didn't put back the fiber.

When it comes to fiber, we mostly think about the kind we are urged to eat for regularity, which is the soluble variety and is found in whole grains such as wheat, rice, and corn. It is the main fiber found in most breakfast cereals.

The American Heart Association urges us to eat 25 grams of fiber—any fiber—every day, because in addition to its nutritional benefits, it makes an excellent substitute for heart-harming fats and sugar foods. Although it doesn't attack cholesterol like oat bran, wheat bran may be better for the heart than originally believed.

A few studies have shown a relationship between a lower risk of cardiovascular disease and consumption of whole grains. The Nurses' Healthy Study, for example, showed that after 10 years,

More Than Fiber

Fiber isn't the whole story when it comes to whole grains. They contain a full complement of nutrients—including B vitamins, phytonutrients, antioxidants, and certain minerals, such as chromium, copper, magnesium, and selenium, that also contribute to heart health. Luckily, most fiber options are not hard to swallow.

those who ate whole grains, including dark bread, brown rice, popcorn, and whole-grain breakfast cereals, had a 30 percent lower risk of heart disease than the nurses who ate refined grains such as white bread, pizza, sweets, and English muffins. But the study's authors noted that the whole-grain-eating nurses also tended to practice other heart-healthy habits, including not smoking.

This does not mean that wheat bran and its cousins should be dismissed as heart-healthy foods. A study of 43,000 men showed results similar to the nurses' study: Those who ate the most whole grains were 30 percent less likely to develop heart disease. Another study in women showed that eating rye and wheat breads helped alleviate the insulin resistance that leads to diabetes.

It's possible that wheat fiber may turn out to have its biggest effect on blood pressure. Researchers from Tulane University in New Orleans examined a large number of studies and found that people with high blood pressure were able to bring it down by eating between 7.2 and 18.9 grams of wheat fiber a day.

Stay away from breakfast candy. Just because a cereal is touted as whole grain does not mean it is healthy. Some whole-grain cereals are 50 percent sugar. That makes them breakfast candy! Keep this in mind: the more sugar, the less grain and fiber. So read labels

---

The Whole Truth

Wheat flour—healthy or not? Not. If a label does not have the word "whole" with the grain, then it is not a whole grain. For example, wheat flour refers to whole-grain wheat that has been refined. The heart-healthy stuff has been taken out of it.

---

carefully. As a rule of thumb, look for cereals that contain at least 3 grams of fiber per serving.

Bran is the leader. This doesn't mean you have to eat bran straight, which many women do not find very appealing. But you should focus on eating breads that are fiber-filled—rye, wheat, or anything that has a lot of texture and is not white. In addition to being full of fiber, they are full of flavor. So take advantage of a good thing!

Kernels of corn. Half the fiber in popcorn is soluble. It is sanctioned as a heart-healthy snack as long as it is air-popped and you forgo the butter.

Tip 25: See That You Get Some Psyllium

No matter how hard we try, some women just can't seem to get enough fiber. If you are one of them, consider a natural fiber-therapy drink. Metamucil, which was part of the Portfolio Diet, and Citrucel are natural laxative drinks that contain soluble fiber from psyllium. They come in different flavors that make them pleasant to drink.

WHAT TO EAT IN PLACE OF MEAT

"My first experience with heart disease was when my father had a heart attack at age 42. I was 14. My second experience was when my father died from a second heart attack. I was 29. My third was when I had a heart attack. I was 51."
— DeArra

The typical American diet favors red meat, deli foods, fried foods, salty snacks, more snacks, fast foods, and soft drinks—often pushed on us in supersize portions. Statistics show that 11 percent of our total fat intake comes from pizza, French fries, cheeseburgers, and burritos. Also, we get 46 percent of our calories from refined white wheat flour and another 24 percent from sugar, both of which do our hearts no favor.

Taking a Big Fat Chance

The Nurses' Health Study gives us a good idea where our unhealthy

---

Meatless Cassoulet

Winter root vegetables replace the traditional meats and sausages in this dish that comes courtesy of cardiologist Sharonne N. Hayes, M.D., of Mayo Clinic. She suggests serving it with whole-grain bread, a simple salad, and red wine.

- 6   **shallots, peeled and quartered**
- 4   **cloves garlic, minced**
- 3   **large carrots, peeled and sliced**
- 1–2 **tablespoons olive oil**
- 1   **turnip, peeled and sliced**
- 1   **parsnip, peeled and chopped**
- 2   **15.5-ounce cans Great Northern beans, drained and rinsed**
- 1   **15.5-ounce can cannelini (white kidney beans) or garbanzo beans (chickpeas)**
- 1   **14.5-ounce can crushed tomatoes (with juice), undrained**

---

eating habits are leading us.

The researchers divided 71,768 nurses with no known heart disease into two groups—Prudent Eaters and Western Eaters—according to how they responded to a food questionnaire.

The Prudent Eaters were identified by their interest in fruits, vegetables, fish, legumes, and whole grains. The Western Eaters were more partial to meat, potatoes, fast foods, and processed foods and didn't go in much for fruits, vegetables, and whole grains. Their diets were monitored for the next 14 years. In the end, the hardiest

1½ **cups chicken or vegetable stock**

2   **bay leaves**

1¼ **teaspoons dried thyme**

    Salt and pepper, to taste

3-4 **slices day-old bread**

2   **tablespoons minced fresh parsley**

In a large Dutch oven, sauté the shallots, garlic, and carrots in the oil over medium heat until soft, about 10 minutes. Lower the heat and add the turnips, parsnips, beans, tomatoes (with juice), stock, bay leaves, thyme, and salt and pepper. Simmer, covered, for about 1 to 1½ hours.

Meanwhile, toast the bread in a 350°F oven for about 10 minutes. Break into crumbs and combine with the parsley. Remove the bay leaves and stir in the bread crumbs before serving.

Serves 4.

Western Eaters had a 58 percent higher risk factor for heart disease and stroke than the meekest Prudent Eaters.

In another study, the Mayo Clinic set out to find the health risks, if any, for 29,000 older women who ate a high-protein diet including red meat and dairy products, such as butter and cheese. After accounting for overweight, smoking, and other risk factors, the researchers found that those who reported the highest intake of these foods increased their risk of dying from heart disease within the next 15 years by 40 percent over those who reported eating the smallest amounts of these foods.

Lead researcher and epidemiologist Dr. Linda E. Keleman said results like this put into question the safety of high-protein diets that emphasize meat and cheese rather than healthful, vegetable-based protein. In fact, the same study found that women who got their protein from foods like beans, nuts, tofu, and peanut butter had a 30 percent lower risk of heart disease than women who ate the least amount of these foods.

Tip 26: Go Meatless for a Day

Being vegetarian has its advantages. Studies show that, on average, vegetarian women are slimmer, have lower blood pressure and cholesterol levels, and are less likely to have a heart attack or stroke than women who eat animal products. This is especially true where blood pressure is concerned. Plant-based foods are rich in potassium, a mineral shown to help regulate blood pressure. On the other

Make an effort to **go meatless** 3 days a week.

hand, women who follow a strict vegetarian diet can, after decades of adherence, end up with vitamin B_{12} and iron deficiencies.

To get some of the extra benefits found only in vegetable-based foods without the risk of deficiencies, nutritionists recommended going vegetarian at least 3 days a week. If that seems like a tall order, start by going meatless 1 day a week and work your way up.

"Substitute a veggie burger for a hamburger tonight and have pasta marinara without meatballs tomorrow night," says Neal Barnard, M.D., who did an analysis of more than 80 studies on the vegetarian lifestyle. "After about 6 weeks of small changes like this, you should notice a drop in blood pressure."

The Queen Bean

Soy is a unique heart protector on several levels. It is the perfect substitute for meat because it contains protein that comes from a plant, meaning it does not contain heart-damaging saturated fat. It is almost complete protein, meaning it contains most of the essential amino acids necessary to build human tissue—a rarity in the plant world. It is chock-full of nutrients, especially vitamin B_6, which has special importance to women's health. Soy is the chief source of special compounds called isoflavones, a type of phytoestrogen—akin to, you guessed it, female estrogen.

Tip 27: Put a Little Soy in Your Life

Studies show that women who eat soy products in place of meat have lower cholesterol levels. An analysis of 38 studies in which soy replaced meat in people's diets found that eating an average of 47

The Story on Salt

Salt's role in heart disease has been an on-again/off-again debate among scientists. But it hasn't made much of an impression on everyone else. If anything, salt consumption has gone up.

Estimates put the average American daily salt consumption between 3,500 and 4,000 milligrams a day. Health standards say we should get no more than 2,400 milligrams a day, and people with high blood pressure who are salt sensitive should limit salt to 1,500 milligrams a day.

Salt's association with high blood pressure is clear. Salt increases water retention, which increases blood volume, which increases the pressure as it flows through the arteries, if it is not excreted. People with high blood pressure may not be able to excrete it sufficiently. Studies of people with high blood pressure have found low salt intake consistent with the lowest blood pressure levels.

The problem is that salt is hard to avoid. It is everywhere. The food industry depends on it because it extends the shelf life of packaged foods and makes the ingredients taste better. It is in our daily staples of bread and milk. It can save a botched-up recipe at the last minute. Some cuisines depend on it to deliver their unique secret flavors.

Most of the salt we get comes from places other than the salt shaker on the kitchen table. This means you should be mindful of salt when buying packaged food for your pantry. Here's the rule from a nutritionist's thumb: Don't buy any product that contains more sodium than calories.

grams of soy protein per day—about 1½ ounces—reduced total cholesterol, LDL cholesterol, and triglycerides without affecting levels of protective HDL cholesterol.

The protein in soy is considered star quality because it has a unique way of binding with the isoflavones that enhance their health power.

The daily dose. You can overdo a good thing. There is some concern among nutritionists and scientists that eating too much soy protein can cause a health-compromising imbalance in women's hormone levels. The Food and Drug Administration says that eating 25 grams of soy protein a day is a safe level and enough to guard against heart disease.

Go for the real thing. Some women just don't like soy and attempt to eat "pretend" hot dogs or bologna made out of soy in the name of health. You'd be better off looking for healthy food elsewhere. Soy dogs and bologna are manufactured just like other processed foods and contain a lot of sodium. Your best bet is to avoid imitation food and stick to the real thing.

Tofu is good for you. Tofu is the chameleon of soy. Unlike other manufactured soy products, it has the unique ability to take on the flavor of other foods it mingles with in a dish. If you tried it in one recipe and didn't like it, try it again. Or if you didn't like the texture, try a firmer or softer variety. Tofu, which is minimally processed, works well as a substitute for meat in many recipes. The valuable isoflavones in tofu deteriorate when heated, though, so add it to

You can eat up to 25 grams a day of **soy protein** as a replacement for **animal protein**.

cooked dishes at the last minute.

Use soy for its protein-added value. Try adding soy to soups, smoothies, or breads. It's a great way to incorporate soy into your diet if you are one of the many women who find soy products tasteless or unappetizing. Be creative and experiment a little in the kitchen to reap the benefits of eating soy.

Eat edamame. These are edible green soybeans that make a delicious and healthful snack. They can be found packaged and ready to pop in your mouth in most good supermarkets.

Check labels. When checking out soy products in the supermarket, read the labels. If soy isn't listed among the first three ingredients, the food doesn't have enough soy to be worth the calories.

Tip 28: Eggs Every Day

. . . and every way, if you so desire, as long as it is part of a low-fat diet. Eggs have more concentrated protein within their little shells than any other food. Eggs are controversial because the yolk of one large egg contains around 200 milligrams of cholesterol—two-thirds of what is considered a healthy daily intake.

It turns out, however, that the cholesterol danger in eggs is not what it's been cracked up to be. One reason is that eggs contain virtually no saturated fat. Three studies—one in Israel and others at Yale and Harvard universities—found that eating eggs every day does not raise cholesterol.

In the Yale study, researchers had adults with normal cholesterol eat eggs daily for 9 weeks. In Israel, one to three eggs were given to people with moderately high cholesterol for 9 weeks. Neither group showed a spike in cholesterol levels as a result of eating the eggs.

"What this means is that you can eat eggs even if you have high cholesterol, but only under two conditions," says Olga Raz, one of the Israeli researchers. "You must keep your saturated fat consumption low, and you must increase your consumption of monounsaturated fat, like olive oil and canola oil."

Bottom line: You can have your eggs any way, as long as you don't make them in butter.

Red Beet Eggs

Hard-cooked eggs make a good snack, but they can get boring. Plus, to stay on the health side, you want to limit eating them to one at a time. Pickled eggs pick up extra flavor, and you fill up by eating the beets, which are rich in folate. This is a recipe passed down from my grandmother.

1	**dozen large eggs**
1	**16-ounce can sliced red beets, with their juice**
¼	**cup brown sugar**
½	**cup cold water**
3-4	**cloves**
¼	**teaspoon cinnamon**

Hard-boil the eggs and let them cool. In a bowl large enough to hold the eggs, add the beets and juice, then stir in the brown sugar, water, cloves, and cinnamon. Peel the eggs and add to the juice. Refrigerate and turn every four hours. They are ready when the eggs turn a deep pink, which takes about a day.

5 What **Color Is** Your Dinner **Plate?**

Women, for the most part, make a good effort to avoid high-fat food. Though we may not be scoring an A, it's a safe bet that many of us are making a solid B. We eat less red meat than we used to, and eat more chicken and fish. In fact, we are way below the national average of 81.4 grams of daily fat intake. The average female eats 67.4 grams a day compared to men, who get 99 grams. Nevertheless, our diets are still too high in fat.

So where are we going wrong? It seems that we are worrying more about what we shouldn't be eating instead of concentrating on what we could and should be enjoying. In short, we are not eating enough fruits and vegetables, our hearts' key protectors against the assaults of daily living. Only a quarter of the women in the United States report eating at least five servings of fruits and vegetables a day—the minimum recommended for heart health by the American Heart Association.

When you read what you're missing out on, you'll see that there are plenty of tasty ways to improve our record.

MOTHER KNOWS BEST

"I owe my recovery from a heart attack to the discipline of eating heart-healthy food and exercise. I'm dedicated to giving my heart a better place to live." — Mary, age 80

It's been decades since science first discovered that certain foods possess unique qualities that can alter body chemistry in ways that can either help or hinder the mechanisms controlling the steady beat of the heart. Though early scientists looked to life-sustaining vitamins and minerals for clues, they now know that certain foods contain other minute compounds that bestow special gifts on the heart. Scientists call these substances phytonutrients, or phytochemicals, and they come courtesy of Mother Nature. Leading the pack are a large family called polyphenols which behave in the body like antioxidants, the armed guards of the heart.

Antioxidants are one of the top reasons why food is such a powerful heart protector. They are crucial workers on the heart's behalf because they target a process called oxidation in which substances known as free radicals accumulate in the body and damage cells. Oxidation is what causes LDL cholesterol to harden and cling to artery walls. Picture a sliced apple that turns the color of rust after it is exposed to air. That's oxidation. If, however, you squirt the exposed flesh with antioxidant-containing lemon juice, it stays white. Antioxidants protect the heart in a similar way. A number of studies have shown a strong association between a high intake of antioxidant foods and a lower incidence of heart disease.

At one time, scientists thought that only the traditional anti-oxidants—vitamin C, vitamin E, beta-carotene (a form of vitamin A), and the mineral selenium—could do the job. Then, more than a decade ago, researchers discovered that plant foods contain a mother lode of other compounds with the potential to unleash a number of healthful benefits. Some have the ability to target processes that clog arteries, lead to blood clots, and produce inflammation. Others help prevent the insulin resistance that leads to type 2 diabetes. Hundreds of these substances so far have been identified in edible plants, most notably subclasses of polyphenols known as phenolic acids, flavonoids, lignans, and stilbenes. All have been found to offer special benefits to the heart.

Tip 29: **Follow the Rainbow**

It was the discovery of polyphenols that led scientists to the conclusion that taking antioxidant supplements such as vitamin E and beta-carotene alone may not be enough to protect your heart. Most of these substances are hidden in a plant's pigment, which is what gives it a distinctive color. In nature, these special nutrients play a protective role for the plant itself. In the body, scientists are now finding they have the potential to protect us from a variety of harmful diseases, like heart disease. Unlike vitamins, which are essential to keep us healthy and alive, we can survive without phytonutrients. Consuming them, however, can bestow benefits science is only beginning to uncover. These nutrients are believed to number in the thousands—most of them yet to be identified—and scientists are

> **What Is a Serving?**
> Five servings seem like a lot. But they are not, if you don't confuse serving size with portion size. For example, a serving size is one small apple or orange, half a grapefruit, or a small salad you would eat as a side dish. Here's another example. A serving size of pasta is a half-cup. How often is your dinner *portion* just one half-cup?

still investigating their full potential. That's why the way to ensure you are getting the best variety is to go for color. Your plate should be a rainbow of blues, greens, reds, and yellows—signs that there is something special in your food.

Nearly all fruits and vegetables fit this color code, which is why we are encouraged to eat lots of them. To list them all, and all their potential, could fill a book. These are among the special ones that should share a plate for your heart.

HUES OF BLUES

> *"My three blocked arteries weren't discovered until my heart failed during surgery for carpal tunnel."* — Martha, age 61

Foods with blue and purple hues belong to a class of phytonutrients called flavonoids and get their color from anthocyanins, pigments that are believed to help support strength in vein walls. They may also enhance the antioxidant action of vitamin C. The deeper the color, the better. Anthocyanins are found closest to the skin and increase with ripeness, so no peeling!

Tip 30: **Enjoy the Blues**

They are mighty tiny, but blueberries are emerging as mighty powerful heart saviors. Researchers at Tufts University analyzed 60 fruits and vegetables for their antioxidant properties and the baby blue came in number one. There is more health in a handful of blues than a bowl of vegetables.

Blueberries are a powerhouse of a compound called pterostilbene, which has the ability to activate the cellular structure that helps lower cholesterol—the same target of cholesterol-lowering drugs. Preliminary studies suggest that blueberries can produce results similar to some of these medications. Blueberries guard against other diseases as well, including diabetes and cancer.

Blueberries also contain a compound called ellagic acid, which works together with anthocyanins to reduce the inflammation in the body that puts the heart at risk. As a bonus, blueberries are brimming with vitamin C and are low in calories.

The daily dose. While blueberries may never become a replacement for cholesterol-lowering drugs, you can eat them to your heart's desire. Blueberry researchers suggest that a cup or two a day is optimal.

Blueberries can be found year-round, thanks to imports from

Aim to eat a minimum of **five servings** of fruits and vegetables in a variety of colors every day.

New Zealand, but the tastiest are the all-American variety, which are in season from May to October. New Jersey has laid claim to being the blueberry capital of the world by declaring it the state fruit. Take advantage of any opportunity to get Jersey blues; in my clearly biased opinion, they taste the best.

Scatter them around. Blueberries are tasty treats eaten alone but they go well with just about everything, from pancakes and muffins to toppings and glazes for chicken and fish and, of course, desserts. Throw a bunch of blueberries on your oatmeal and whole-grain cereals at breakfast. Blueberries are so versatile that an entire cookbook is devoted to them. *True Blueberry*, by Linda Dannenberg, is loaded with great ideas and great recipes.

Tip 31: Go by Skin Tone

Though the blue is the queen berry, all plant foods with a blue or purple skin tone contain anthocyanins. Blackberries and black currants, in particular, contain a high concentration. They are also a very special taste treat.

SHADES OF RED

> *"One January morning, I woke up at 8:00 a.m. and decided to quit smoking. At 4:00 p.m., I had a heart attack."*
> — Susan, age 41

Reds and oranges are symbols of heart health. Anthocyanins, which put the blue in blueberries, are also responsible for imparting the colorful skin in rich red fruits. But the real superstar is a nutrient known as beta-carotene, a member of a powerful class of anti-oxidants that convert into an active form of vitamin A (retinol) in the body. The rich, deep color that goes clean into the flesh of some vegetables, like carrots and sweet potatoes, is a sign that this super-nutrient is well-represented.

Tip 32: Mix a Bowl of Berries

It's no wonder the strawberry is shaped like a heart. Strawberries are rich in polyphenols but their anthocyanin content, unlike in other fruits, extends into the flesh. They also overflow with vitamin C—1 cup offers 141 percent of the recommended daily value.

Raspberries contain only half the powerful vitamin C content of strawberries, but they make up for it in fiber. A cup of raspberries

---

Simply Delicious

Red raspberries are synonymous with the phrase "simply delicious!" Raspberry sauce is a well-known topping for desserts, but it is also great atop grilled chicken and turkey. Just thaw out a bag of frozen berries and put them, undrained, in a food processor until smooth. Serve at room temperature spooned over grilled poultry.

For a smoother topping, you can purge the seeds from the juice by pushing the berries through a mesh strainer with the back of a spoon. You'll get an entirely different texture and flavor, but by extracting the seeds, you also lose the fiber.

---

contains 6 grams of dietary fiber.

Both raspberries and strawberries are a rare source of the polyphenol called ellagic acid, which is not found in many edible plant foods.

Fresh is best. You'll get the most out of their vitamin C by eating berries fresh. Eat them with whole-grain cereals or mix them into a bowl of low-fat vanilla yogurt for a refreshing snack or light lunch—and an extra shot of health.

Cherry-Flavored Protection?

Cherries have long been reputed to help ward off a gout attack, but preliminary research indicates that they may help lower the risk of a future heart attack and stroke.

Cherries are known as an anti-gout food because they help break up uric acid crystals in joints, usually in the big toe, that cause pain and swelling. Crystals form when concentrations of uric acid are high. Many of the foods that cause a buildup of uric acid also happen to be foods that cause heart trouble down the line, like beef and organ meats. This made researchers wonder if there could be a link between high uric acid buildup and a future date with heart trouble or stroke.

To test the theory, University of California researchers had 10 women with normal uric acid levels eat 45 cherries each and then tested their uric acid. Levels dropped 15 percent. If further research proves a link between uric acid and heart disease, a bowlful of cherries could be a safety net.

The researchers determined that any kind of cherries will do, even maraschinos, and that as little as a handful a day may offer protection.

Tender treatment. Raspberries are highly perishable so eat them as soon as possible after picking or purchasing them. Select berries that are firm and plump. Before putting them in the refrigerator, make sure you remove any that are moldy or have been damaged.

Raspberries freeze well, and it will not harm their nutrients. Wash them, place them in a single layer on a baking sheet, and put them in the freezer. Once the berries are frozen, you can gather them and put them in plastic freezer bags for more permanent storage.

Strawberries are not as delicate, but you get the maximum freshness out of them by hulling and washing them right before you use them. Many people like to pop a fresh strawberry right into their mouths. Put some in a plastic sandwich bag and take them to work for a quick and healthy morning or afternoon snack.

Caution. Strawberries and raspberries are among a small number of foods that contain high amounts of oxalic acid, which can be a problem for people prone to gallstones and kidney stones. They are also a common food allergen.

Tip 33: **Count on the Cranberry**

Women have been drinking cranberry juice for decades as a natural remedy to prevent and help cure urinary tract infections. There is now evidence that it is also qualified to assist the heart.

Cranberries are an excellent source of pterostilbene, the same compound in blueberries that helps fight cholesterol. One study found that drinking three glasses of cranberry juice a day did not affect harmful LDL cholesterol, but it did increase protective HDL cholesterol by 10 percent.

Good news: cholesterol-fighting cranberries come in season about

Berry Fruity Chutney

This chutney is brimming with so many nutrients it's like heart armor! It goes with just about anything—poultry, pork, fish—or serve it as a dip for celery or pita bread.

1	tablespoon olive oil
¼	cup chopped shallot
1	bag (12 ounces) fresh cranberries
1	ripe papaya, seeded
½	cup orange juice
2	tablespoons cider vinegar
2	tablespoons minced cilantro
¼	cup chopped walnuts
	Salt and black pepper, to taste
	Ground red pepper, to taste

Heat the oil in a medium saucepan and sauté the shallots until soft, but not brown. Add the cranberries, papaya, orange juice, and vinegar. Bring to a boil. Lower the heat and simmer until the cranberries are soft and pop, about 10 minutes. Remove from the heat and cool slightly. Add the cilantro, walnuts, and seasonings. Cover and refrigerate until ready to use.

Makes about 3 cups.

the same time that the berries of summer are just about gone.

Dump the mayo. Make a fresh cranberry relish as a substitute topping for mayonnaise on turkey and chicken sandwiches. Process a bag of fresh berries with a few oranges in a food processor until smooth. Add ¼ to ½ cup of sugar and let the mixture macerate for a few days in the refrigerator. You'll get a not-too-sweet relish that will keep in the refrigerator for a few weeks.

Tip 34: Try Tomatoes, Any Style

If you're seeing more men in pizza parlors and Italian restaurants lately, they may be trying to fill up on tomatoes, the vegetable being widely publicized as a superfood for prostate health. They may not realize it, but they also are doing their hearts a big favor. That means you should be taking advantage of Italian fare, too.

The crown jewel of the tomato is a carotenoid called lycopene, the substance believed to be beneficial to both the prostate and the heart. But lycopene is only one of many substances that make tomatoes guardians of the heart. They are rich in the unique phytonutrient called flavonol, plus they contain vitamin A, vitamin C, folate, and the mineral potassium, all of which protect the heart in special ways. Folate is the focus of heart health because it helps reduce high levels of homocysteine, an amino acid associated with an increased risk for heart attack and stroke. Potassium helps keep blood pressure in check. Researchers suspect that synergy among all these nutrients helps enhance the tomato's protective action.

Tomatoes are a sun-kissed staple of the Mediterranean and another testament to the healthfulness of the region's diet. But you don't have to eat tomatoes ripe from the vine to get their health benefits. Tomatoes in any form are just as beneficial, according to several studies involving women.

One study, conducted at Brigham and Women's Hospital in Boston, followed the tomato consumption of nearly 40,000 middle-age and older women with no known heart disease. After a 7-year follow-up, researchers found that those who consumed 7 to 10 servings a week of lycopene-rich tomato products had a cardio-vascular disease risk 29 percent lower than women who ate 1½

Folate: The Mom's Vitamin

Mothers are no strangers to folate. They need to be mindful of it before and during early pregnancy to guard against birth defects, and after pregnancy for the growth of a new infant. We now have another reason to make sure we get enough of this B vitamin: It's good for the heart.

Researchers have found a link between high folate levels and a reduced risk of heart attack. Folate is important because it helps purge excess levels of homocysteine, an amino acid researchers believe contributes to the buildup of artery-clogging plaque. Though it is still not known for sure if lowering homocysteine levels lowers the risk for heart disease, nutritionists say eating high-folate foods is a good idea.

Here is another reason to eat folate: It can help reduce blood pressure. An analysis of more than 62,000 middle-age and older women in the Nurses' Health Study found that those who consumed at least 1,000 micrograms a day (the recommended daily value is 400) had a 46 percent reduced risk of developing high blood pressure. Other studies found similar results.

Folate is naturally present in a lot of foods, and many packaged foods, like cereal, are enriched with it. You can also find folate in most of the fruits and vegetables discussed in this chapter. Nutritionists say, however, that the best way to absorb it is from a supplement. A multivitamin tablet contain-ing 400 micrograms should be adequate.

servings or less a week. Here's something even more interesting: Women who ate oil-based tomato products, even pizza, had a 34 percent reduced risk. This is because more lycopene is absorbed when it is dissolved in fat, notably olive oil, says Olga Raz, R.D., a nutrition researcher from Israel.

Choose the little ones. Beefsteaks may win the size prize but grape tomatoes get the best of show. Flavonol biosynthesis is stimulated by light, meaning the nutrient accumulates in the outer skin. The skin can contain as much as ten times more flavonol than the flesh, meaning that, bite for bite, cherry tomatoes are top dog.

Seeds and all. Whether fresh or canned, use the tomato for all its worth. Studies show whole tomatoes are nutritionally superior to skinned-and-seeded varieties. In fact, a preliminary study in Scotland suggests that the seeds themselves may contain a compound that helps prevent blood clots. The study, conducted at the Rowett Research Institute in Aberdeen, found that people who drank a special tomato juice containing the seeds and its gel-like casing reduced the potential for blood clots by 72 percent. So, when a recipe calls for peeling and seeding a tomato, be a rebel and throw in the whole thing.

No need to be fussy. Sauce, paste, ketchup, juice, soup. It appears any kind of tomato product has health benefits. However, many of these products contain lots of salt and preservatives, so if these are off your diet by doctor's orders, then they are not for you.

Cook and enhance. Carotenoids are enhanced through cooking, especially with added olive oil, so boil away.

Summer advantage. Eating doesn't get any better than a summer tomato, red and ripe off the vine. For the most taste and nutrition, let color be your guide.

Go for gazpacho. Researchers at Tufts University put gazpacho,

Gazpacho

The ingredients make for one cholesterol-kicking soup!

2½	pounds summer-ripe tomatoes, chopped
1	green bell pepper, seeded and diced
1	yellow bell pepper, seeded and diced
1	small red onion, diced
1	cup tomato juice
¼	cup red wine vinegar
2	tablespoons extra-virgin olive oil
1	jalapeño pepper, seeded and minced
½	teaspoon salt

Add all the ingredients to a food processor. Give it four or five quick on-and-off spins. Put the soup in a bowl and chill for at least 2 hours before serving.

Note: When handling jalapeños, wash your hands thoroughly afterward. They can give your eyes quite a sting if your hands get near your face.

Serves 4.

a tomato-based uncooked soup, to the test and found it had heart-protecting qualities. The people in the study ate two bowlfuls a day for 2 weeks.

Tip 35: Explore the Oranges

Orange is the color of nutritional wealth. Carrots, pumpkin, and sweet potatoes are the most common and the tastiest standouts. Keep the sweet potato in mind when you are hankering for a starchy side dish. Other potatoes pale in its presence. Sweets are particularly rich in carotenoids. In addition to its heart benefit, at least one study showed that the sweet potato contains a substance that can help regulate blood sugar.

A good mash. Bake sweet potatoes until soft and boil carrots in water until tender. After the potatoes cool, peel them and mash them with the carrots. Add a teaspoon or two of olive oil and some chopped nuts. Put in a casserole and reheat for a dinner side dish.

Tip 36: **Dare to Do Onions**

Onions stand out in the vegetable patch as one of the richest sources of flavonol. Onions are also the richest source and one of the few foods that contains hydroxybenzoic acid, a special type of phytonutrient that makes its antioxidant power even stronger. Studies have found that eating onions can help bring down cholesterol, lower blood pressure, and help regulate blood sugar.

A study in India found that people who ate the most onions, about a pound a week, had lower cholesterol levels than those who didn't eat any onions. In another study, researchers purposely raised the cholesterol in a group of men by having them eat half a stick of butter a day as part of their normal diet. No surprise: Their cholesterol went up. They then added 2 ounces of raw onion juice to their daily serving of butter. The result: The onion juice slowed a second rise in cholesterol.

Eat them in the raw. Onions contain a healthy substance called quercetin, which is rare in edible plants. The compound, however, dissipates when cooked, so you will only get the benefit of this heart-healthy compound when you eat onions raw.

The stronger, the better. Onions get their pungent taste and smell from sulfur. When onions were evaluated for their nutrient density, researchers found a correlation between high-sulfur and high-nutrient content. Yellow onions are the strongest and Vidalia onions, which are grown in Georgia, are the sweetest and mildest.

Use steam heat. When cooking onions, forget the butter and sauté onions in a little olive or canola oil. To keep the onions from soaking up too much oil (and adding extra calories you don't need), lower the heat and cover them with a tight lid. You'll end up with crunchy but not greasy onions.

It's all in the family. Leeks, shallots, and scallions are all part of the onion family and deliver similar benefits. Shallots pack a particularly good punch. Bite for bite, they contain more than twice the phytonutrients of a Vidalia onion.

THE GREEN GIANTS

> "I'm 21 with a cholesterol level of 360, and my HDLs
> are only 32.My dad died of a misdiagnosed heart attack at
> 46. This worries me, so I went to see a cardiologist.
> He told me to come back when I'm 40!" — Kellie

If it's green, it's good for you—right? We've been hearing that since we stared down that first plate of peas when we were about age 3. Not only was mom's advice good but, through the years, we have grown fond of greens. Often, we'll forgo a burger and fries in favor of a mixed-greens salad at lunch.

Leafy greens are the most ubiquitous vegetables in the marketplace, and our choices of salad fixings have grown a lot in the last 10 years. That makes for good adventure in eating, but it is not always easy to figure out where the various greens stand nutritionally. To be a good greens keeper, you need to know where to aim your fork. Here are some guidelines.

Tip 37: **Go for the Dark and Curly**

Like code orange, dark green is a signal that beta-carotene is somewhere inside. Even the much-maligned iceberg lettuce has some nutritional value, as long as you stay away from the heart and nibble on the darker outer leaves. Phytochemicals are so called because their biosynthesis is stimulated by light (phyto). Important flavonoids are concentrated in the outer layer of leaves. Curly greens like kale and romaine lettuce can hold as much as 10 times more nutritional value in the leaves that feel the warmth of the sun than in the leaves found in the pale inner core. They also contain folate, vitamin C, beta-carotene, and potassium as well as phytonutrients and carotenoids.

The lettuce family is huge, and new and more peculiar offshoots are cropping up all the time. So, go for it. If it's green, clean, and crisp, you won't venture out of the heart zone.

Tip 38: **Make Romaine Home Plate**

Not all greens are lettuces—but why get technical? Keep it simple and use commonly found romaine lettuce as a base for building a salad. You'll know the leaves are fresh and crisp if they yield a tad of milky liquid when broken. Break them up, throw them in a bowl, and go color crazy with the rest of the ingredients. Your imagination is the limit. Add vegetables, fruits, and even leftover lean meat. It's a great way to make use of leftovers.

Tip 39: **Always Dress Sensibly**

The only way you can really go wrong with a salad is by going overboard on the dressing. Even if you use heart-healthy olive oil, you are still getting about 120 calories a tablespoon. Olive oil is a heart food but it is not a diet food!

Toss it around. Salad doesn't need as much dressing as you might think. If you toss it in a large bowl so the ingredients have room to actually move, the oil will lightly coat the leaves just as it should. Olive oil has a powerful taste, and a little goes a long way. If you just plop the dressing on top of a salad already plated, you will unnecessarily add too much salad dressing, soak the leaves, and boost your calorie content. It is worth the extra time and dishes to do it right.

Tip 40: **Beware of Caesar Salad**

When ordering out, beware of getting caught in a fat trap. Restaurants that offer giant chicken- or shrimp-topped Caesar salads in the name of health are not always doing your waistline a favor. It is not uncommon for a restaurant to use an entire head of Romaine lettuce glistening with oil and covered in cheese for a single-serving main dish salad. Figure in the dressing, meat or seafood, cheese, and croutons and you're stepping on the calorie scale. Greek salads and chef salads are even worse. Behind-the-scenes nutritional analyses have measured lunchtime "light" salad meals close to 1,000 calories.

Here are a few strategies for keeping your salad out of the caloric danger zone:

- ♥ If the restaurant serves large salads, split one with a dining partner, or request a half portion.

- ♥ Forget the meat or seafood topping. Since the salad is already large, you don't need the extra food.

- ♥ Asking for dressing on the side kind of defeats the idea of Caesar salad. Instead ask for the croutons and cheese on the side.

- ♥ Eat half of the salad and take the rest home

- ♥ If you are craving a chef salad, ask what kinds of meat and cheese the chef uses. Pass on the ham and salami. Ask for the cheese on the side, take a little and send the rest back with the server.

- ♥ If you want a Greek salad, ask what the chef adds to make it "Greek." Select as you would for a chef salad. Also, ask for the feta and meat on the side.

Tip 41: **Stand by Broccoli**

Broccoli gets healthy raves on many levels, but it is key to heart health because it is one of the richest sources of flavonols. This distinction makes broccoli stand out as one of the few vegetables with the strength to *significantly* help reduce the risk of heart disease. Plus, it also contains folate, vitamin C, potassium, and calcium.

Steam it lightly. Broccoli is hearty, plentiful, inexpensive, and goes with just about anything, making it a standby for everyday meals. It gets much of its power from a substance called quercetin, which loses its nutritional value when cooked. Instead, steam broccoli lightly and you will retain much of the quercetin.

The younger, the better. Young broccoli exudes the most flavor and the most nutrients. For a total taste experience, eat it raw. Also, look for broccoli sprouts at the market. The sprouts contain the most nutrients of all.

Tip 42: Take This Spear to Heart

Only those with a real gift for gardening can truly appreciate the arrival of asparagus. It takes three years of backyard patience to reap the first crop, but home growers get the special privilege of eating it the moment it shoots from the earth, when it is the most tender, succulent, and nutritious. The green spear's biggest claim to heart health is its robust quantity of vitamin A and folate.

Before the days when vegetables were available year-round, asparagus was part of the rite of spring. To many people, it is still considered a delicacy.

Asparagus may be fussy to grow, but figuring out what to do with it is easy. It is extremely versatile. It can be eaten raw, steamed, sautéed, roasted, and grilled. It can be a stand-alone dish or a side dish, and it partners just as well with pasta as it does with steak. It also makes a great soup.

Asparagus tips. The only thing asparagus doesn't do well is stay fresh. Asparagus should be eaten within a day or two of picking or purchasing. Look for stalks that stand tall with tips that are tight, firm, and colorful. Chefs prefer fatter spears over the thin. To preserve its precious folate content, wrap the asparagus in a damp paper towel and store it in the back of the refrigerator so it is away from the light. Folate doesn't fair well when exposed to light, air, or heat.

Tip 43: Give Spinach the Thumbs Up

Maybe spinach would have made a better impression on us if Olive Oyl, rather than Popeye, had devoured it by the canful. Popeye tried to push spinach on us because of its iron content, but, the truth is, most of the blood-building iron in spinach isn't absorbed very well by the body. But its female-friendly, blood-boosting folate content is absorbed very well, and spinach contains plenty of it. It also is an excellent source of vitamin A, vitamin C, the mineral potassium, polyphenols, and carotenoids. Plus, it is a rich source of magnesium, which, like potassium, helps keep blood pressure in check. That gives spinach a 5-star rating for heart health.

Most studies on spinach and heart health have focused on its ability to help reduce blood pressure. One study, conducted on rats, showed a reduction in blood pressure within a few hours after eating spinach. The same effect, according to the researchers, could be achieved in humans by eating a large spinach salad.

There doesn't appear to be much difference if you buy spinach fresh or frozen (or in a can, like Popeye), but fresh wins in the taste category.

Tip 44: **Pick Peppers – Sweet and Hot**

You can make a colorful plate using nothing but bell peppers! They come in vivid shades of green, red, yellow, orange, and even purple—all colors that advertise that they are rich in carotenoids and anti-oxidant vitamins. They are also a good source of folate.

Red peppers offer a bonus the other colors don't. They are a rare source of lycopene, the substance that makes tomatoes so healthy. That's good news for pimiento lovers, too. The green variety is a rare source of heart-healthy quercetin and phytosterols. But no matter what color you choose, you can be sure you'll get good nutrition, especially vitamin C.

Some people find sweet bells as well as hot peppers hard on the stomach. Also, there are those who will argue that peppers are an acquired taste, especially when it comes to hot peppers. But it is worth developing a taste for hot peppers. They are the only peppers that contain capsaicin, the fiery substance that helps lower cholesterol (and has other health benefits as well). The sweet varieties lack the gene responsible for putting the sting in hot peppers.

GRAZING THROUGH THE SUN BELT

"For 2 years after my heart attack, I'd burst into tears at meal-time because I was never sure what I could or should eat."
— Anne, age 48

In sunny climes, you could say, health literally grows on trees. Mediterranean regions like the South of France, Italy, and Greece may be known for creating rich pastries, but what the people really enjoy for dessert day in and day out is no-frills, homegrown fruit. You don't have to live near the Mediterranean among tropical fruit trees to do the same. A variety of fruits, extending to the exotics, are now commonplace in American markets.

Here is a basic rule of thumb: If it comes from a warm climate and grows on a tree, you can assume that it is offering you a good dose of antioxidant vitamin C. Certain fruits offer other benefits for the heart as well. Here are some fruits to keep in mind when you're cruising the produce aisle.

Tip 45: Eat from the Fruit of the Citrus Tree

Citrus stands out in the fruit world as the only rich source of a special compound called flavanones, which have been found to inhibit the formation of blood clots and help lower cholesterol. Flavanones give citrus its bitter taste.

The Fruit Spread

The best way to fit fruit into your lifestyle is to eat it in small amounts as part of a meal or as a snack, recommends Olga Raz, R.D. This is especially important if you have borderline or high blood sugar. Fruit contains fructose, a naturally-occurring sugar. "But it is sugar nonetheless," she says. "The sugar in fruit should not be a problem as long as you do not eat a lot of it in one serving."

Oranges are extra special. Television jingles have been reminding us for decades that a single orange contains more than 100 percent of our recommended daily requirement for vitamin C. Here is

Heart-Healthy Herbs

Herbs have been used as food and medicine for centuries, but it has been only decades since modern scientists validated many of the ancient beliefs about the healing power of plants, including those that contribute to cardiovascular health.

Adding to the healing potential of herbs are more recent discoveries that certain herbs contain a variety of phytochemicals including flavonoids, carotenoids, and plant sterols.

The only problem with herbs is that you eat them in tiny amounts, so you can't really depend on them to supply you with enough nutrients to nurse your heart to health. But you can take advantage of them kind of as a value-added bonus.

Many of the following are made into tea, some help enhance recipes, and some you will find in some of the aromatherapy ideas suggested later in this book. They all contain one or several substances that are good for your heart. Get familiar with these herbs so you can use them when the opportunity arises. They include:

- ♥ Chamomile
- ♥ Dandelion
- ♥ Fenugreek
- ♥ Ginkgo
- ♥ Green tea leaves
- ♥ Hawthorn
- ♥ Juniper berries
- ♥ Lemongrass
- ♥ Mint
- ♥ Parsley
- ♥ Passionflower
- ♥ Onion
- ♥ Rose hips
- ♥ Rosemary
- ♥ Sage
- ♥ Thyme
- ♥ Yarrow

some not-so-common knowledge: A single orange contains more than 160 different kinds of polyphenols and 60 different flavonoids, many of which have cholesterol-lowering potential. Oranges also stand out among the citrus set as a rare source of the compound hesperitin, which can help lower blood pressure and cholesterol.

Get into the pink. You'll get something extra out of grapefruit by choosing the pink and red varieties. They contain lycopene, the nutrient that makes tomatoes a nutritional standout.

Eat the whole thing. The peel and white membranes that form the sections of citrus fruit contain the highest levels of flavanones (called lemonines). For example, you'll get five times the amount of flavanones from eating the fruit than from drinking a glass of orange juice. Though no one would ever expect you to make eating orange peels a habit, you should take advantage of eating the white membranes along with the flesh. Orange, lemon, and lime peels, called the zest, are often recommended additions to recipes. Try adding some zest to some of your own recipes.

Think before you drink. Orange juice, that is. This is not to say you should never touch the stuff, just keep in mind that one glass of orange juice contains almost twice the calories of an orange, and you also miss out on the fiber. Plus, the vitamin C in juice degrades quickly. For the best juice, squeeze your own. It not only tastes better but you avoid the sugar that comes with processed juices. Hint: As the vitamin C content degrades, so does the flavor.

Tip 46: Eat Avocados, Hold the Guilt

When you think of an avocado, does your mind register "sinfully delicious food?" Women seem to be programmed to think of avocados as a can't-have food because of their high-calorie and off-the-charts fat content. If you are counting calories, the first concern has some merit. But the 86-percent fat calories found in every 320-calorie medium avocado are from oleic acid, a monounsaturated fat that is about as good as it gets.

In one study, people with moderately high cholesterol ate avocados every day for a week. After only 7 days, their LDL cholesterol dropped and their protective HDL increased an amazing 11 percent.

Monos aren't the only thing avenging this golden-green fruit. Avocados contain 60 percent more potassium than the highly touted banana, and they are high in folate, fiber, and vitamin C. So do not discount the avocado as a heart-healthy food.

Say si, si to guacamole. This dish gets a bad rap as a fattening food, but it's unjustified. The ingredients—avocados, tomatoes, onions, citrus juice, jalapeño peppers—are all heart-healthy foods. There is nothing in guacamole that is it bad for you. The trouble comes from eating it with corn or tortilla chips. Scoop it up with pita bread instead or use it as a condiment on sandwiches.

Pair it up. You can enjoy an avocado and be mindful of calories by pairing it with other foods. Its most notable partners are chicken, crabmeat, lobster, shrimp, eggs, papaya, and tomato. Add a slice of avocado to a sandwich or put it in a salad. Mash it and eat it on bread. Experiment with ways to make a little go a long way. Note, however, that avocado turns bitter when cooked, so if you are including it in a cooked meal, add it at the very end.

Tip 47: Get a Taste of the Islands

Tropical fruit makes for adventurous and intensely flavored eating.

Plus, tropical fruits have two important things in common: lots of vitamin C and fiber.

The orange flesh of the papaya and mango, for example, are brimming with beta-carotene, as their flesh suggests. They also contain flavonoids and folate. The brilliantly green flesh within the fuzzy brown shell of the kiwi is an unusual source of all three antioxidant vitamins: A, C, and E. These are considered among the most exotic fruits.

The brilliant orange flesh of the more familiar apricot offers a special dose of lycopene. And bananas in their yellow jackets are an excellent source of potassium.

Whatever you select, you can't go wrong eating tropical fruit as long as you eat it in moderation, just as you should with other fruit. So experiment with these colorful exports and enjoy.

Tropical Fruit Salsa

When 82-year-old Polly Lehman came back to work after taking "a little break" for quadruple heart bypass surgery, her chef son wanted to make sure she ate healthy. So every evening, John would cook Mother a special meal that was not part of the regular fare at Mom Chaffe's, an Italian bistro they co-own in West Reading, Pennsylvania. So many patrons asked about the dishes they saw Polly eating that John featured some of them as nightly specials. Polly's favorite was grilled chicken with Tropical Fruit Salsa. This salsa is also good with salmon.

- 3 **tablespoons rice wine vinegar**
- 2 **tablespoons brown sugar**
  Juice of 2 large limes
- 1 **ripe pineapple, peeled, cored, and chopped**
- 2 **ripe mangoes, peeled, seeded, and chopped**
- 1 **red bell pepper, seeded and diced**
- 2 **bunches of scallions, chopped**
- 1 **jalapeño pepper, seeded and chopped (optional)**
- ¼ **cup chopped fresh cilantro, or to taste**

Put the vinegar, brown sugar, and lime juice in a medium saucepan and cook until the sugar dissolves, about 1 minute. Add the pineapple, mangoes, bell peppers, scallions, and jalapeño pepper, if using. Cover and simmer until tender, about 20 minutes. Remove from the heat, stir in the cilantro, and let the salsa cool. Refrigerate until read to use. Serve a few tablespoons over chicken or fish.

Makes about 3 cups.

6 Be Fit, Be **Active**

If doctors were able to give you just one piece of advice about what is best for your heart, they would say: Be active. That's because regular exercise can correct more wrongs and it can do so better than any other heart-smart pursuit. For women who have had a heart attack, being physically active has special significance. It counts big time in reducing their risk of having another one.

No matter what your size, shape, weight, or age, the health of your heart is strongly dependent on how active you are. "If you want a healthy heart, there is nothing more powerful than being physically fit," says Sharonne N. Hayes, M.D., Director of the Women's Heart Clinic at Mayo Clinic in Rochester, Minnesota.

On the other hand, the consequences of being inactive are major. A sedentary lifestyle is just as bad for the heart as smoking or having high cholesterol or high blood pressure, according to the American Heart Association. Research on women at the University of Florida College of Medicine in Gainesville indicates that physical inactivity may even be a bigger risk for a heart attack than obesity.

These are ominous facts when you consider that 70 percent of American women do not exercise on a regular basis, and 41 percent report they are not active at all. Even more distressing to doctors is research showing that the number of women who exercise regularly is going down instead of going up. That's because they know that physical fitness can be a life-saver.

This was demonstrated recently by researchers at Johns Hopkins University in Baltimore who measured the fitness levels of 3,000 women ages 30 to 80 and followed their heart health for an average of 20 years. Overall, those whose physical fitness was below average were 3½ times more likely to die of heart disease than the women who scored above average. But another finding is what really set off

Inactivity: A Teen Trend

Statistics show that only 52 percent of high-school girls are enrolled in physical education classes and only half of them attend fitness classes daily. Among pre-teens, 61.5 percent do not participate in any organized after-school or weekend physical activity.

By the time a girl reaches age 16 or 17, 31 percent of white and 56 percent of black teenagers do not participate in any kind of after-school physical activities. The American Heart Association notes the parallel between these statistics and the rise in overweight and increase in smoking among teen girls.

alarms: Women who had below-average fitness, but were considered at low risk for heart disease, were 13 times more likely to die of heart disease than women who scored above average for fitness. Overall, death rate increased as fitness levels decreased.

The researchers considered two measurements as key: The amount of physical activity the women could sustain safely, based on a standard treadmill test, and the amount of time it took their heart rates to return to normal.

The treadmill test is significant because nearly two-thirds of women who succumb to a sudden death heart attack have had no previous heart-related symptoms, reported the research team. Further, reported Samia Mora, M.D., the study suggests that women may benefit from higher fitness levels even without positive changes in weight or blood pressure and cholesterol levels.

BENEFITS YOU CAN'T DENY

"I must make the decision every day to exercise, even though I am tired. I understand that I must continue the healthy lifestyle I have chosen and maintain it for the rest of my life."
— Odelinda, age 56

Intuitively, we know that we should exercise. We know it will make us feel better and look better. We know it can reduce stress and make everyday tasks seem a whole lot easier "I tell women it is the only action we take against risk factors in which we can actually *feel* the difference. Exercise makes us feel better," says Dr. Hayes.

"Lowering your cholesterol won't make you feel better. Reducing your blood pressure won't make you feel better. Exercise, though maybe not at first, will make you feel better."

Women who show up at Mayo Clinic with heart problems are often surprised to find out just how powerful fitness can be and how many tangible benefits it provides. For example, studies show that regular exercise:

- ♥ Improves the working capacity of the heart by easing the burden on the arteries and veins and reducing heart rate.

- ♥ Can regulate blood pressure by helping to reduce the systolic measure (the top number), meaning the heart muscle will contract with less effort.

- ♥ Contributes to weight loss and helps maintain ideal weight but, most important, helps to whittle the middle.

Keeping your waistline below 35 inches is a major key to preventing heart trouble.

♥ Can regulate blood sugar—essential if you have diabetes or pre-diabetes.

♥ Helps increase all-important HDL cholesterol and lower triglyceride levels.

♥ Improves your sex life. One study at the University of Arkansas in Fayetteville found that young women who exercised four to five times a week rated their sexual performance as above average or better.

♥ Is a potent stress releaser.

♥ Can reduce the symptoms of depression by as much as 50 percent. One study on women found that regular aerobic exercise can be as effective as antidepressants. This is important for women who have had a heart attack, because depression is a common side effect.

Young at Heart

It doesn't matter what age you are now. Your level of physical fitness determines if your heart will be strong enough to help you live actively and independently in your later years.

Researchers in London found that starting a regular exercise program, even in midlife, helps improve quality of life in old age. They followed 6,398 people ages 39 to 63 who either exercised moderately for 2½ hours a week or strenuously for 1½ hours a week and found that everyone, even those with chronic health problems, was fit enough to maintain their independence into old age.

A Johns Hopkins' study measured the effect of exercise on a group of men and women ages 55 to 75 with diagnosed metabolic syndrome, the name given to a cluster of heart disease risks that increases the potential for a heart attack. Participants were put on a regimen of moderate exercise for 60 minutes three times a week. After 6 months, their aerobic fitness improved 16 percent, their strength was enhanced by 17 percent, and abdominal fat diminished by an average of 20 percent. Metabolic syndrome was alleviated in 41 percent.

A study at Northwestern University in Chicago followed 4,400 men and women between the ages of 18 and 30 for 15 years. It found that as levels of fitness rose, risk factors for heart disease dropped. "The key point," reported the researchers, "is that the development of risk factors for heart disease and stroke isn't just the natural result of aging."

Tip 48: Get on the Move

Think of exercise as a 401K program for the heart. The more you put in, the better off you will be in the future. It doesn't take much to enroll—just two legs, a comfortable pair of shoes, and 30 minutes a day. Make a daily deposit and you'll be vested in no time.

The Centers for Disease Control and Prevention and the American College of Sports Medicine agree that 30 minutes of moderately intense exercise every day is all it takes to reduce your risk of heart disease. Intense, however, means heart-pumping exercise—the kind that increases your heart rate for a significant amount of time. It's what doctors call a cardio workout. For the average woman, that means walking at a brisk pace of 3 to 4 miles an hour, or 1½ to 2 miles, in about a half-hour every day.

"If you're walking along and can carry on a regular conversation, that's not cardio," says Dr. Hayes. "If you're huffing and puffing so much that you can't even speak, then you are walking too fast and overdoing it. You should be able to speak, but not comfortably carry on a conversation."

Get your rate right. Your best rate of return on your energy investment is one that gets your heart pumping at just the right speed. Go too slow and it's not cardio. Go too fast and you'll run out of wind. Quit too soon and essentially you'll blow the whole effort. Worse, putting a sudden overdose of stress on the heart can be dangerous.

What's really nice about maintaining your target heart rate is that it doesn't take as much effort as you might think. It is a pace that actually feels comfortable. But then, that's the whole idea.

Your personal target heart rate is dependent on your current conditioning, which means everyone is a little bit different. Doctors, however, have developed a widely used formula, based on age, that

See Your Doctor First

If you are out of shape, age 50 or older, or are being treated for heart disease or any other health condition, you should consult with your physician before starting an exercise program. But do not be timid about starting an exercise program if you have known risk factors. "Women at the highest risk will get the most benefit from exercise," says Sharonne N. Hayes, M.D.

is easy to follow. Subtract your age from 220. This is your maximum heart rate. Your target heart rate zone is between 60 and 75 percent of your maximum.

For example, if you are 50 years old, your maximum heart rate is 170 beats per minute and your target heart rate zone is between 102 and 127 beats per minute. If you're 40, your maximum heart rate is 180 and your target zone is between 108 and 135.

To measure your heart rate, find your pulse by placing your index and middle finger on the thumb side of your wrist and press lightly. Count the number of beats in 10 seconds and multiply by 6. Walk slowly while checking your heart rate.

Measuring heart-rate zone is optional, says Dr. Hayes. If you are not comfortable staying in your zone, or find the whole idea of tracking your target zone too bothersome, simply use the "talk test," she advises.

Tip 49: **Take 10 Anytime**

Where will you find the time? It is a familiar refrain for many women and one doctors hear all the time. You don't have to do 30 minutes in one shot if you don't have the time. You can do 10 minutes at a time three times a day and still get a cardio workout. One small study at Southwest Missouri State University in Springfield found that three 10-minute bursts of exercise can be just as effective as one 30-minute session. And it doesn't mean three clothing changes and showers.

Ten minutes could mean a brisk walk over your lunch hour and another after dinner. It could be a walk up or down 10 flights of stairs if you live or work in a high-rise, or skipping rope while watch-

Cardio Rehab Is the Place to Be

If you have had a heart attack, it is not a good idea to just go walking off on your own. It is imperative that your doctor be your exercise guide, says Sharonne N. Hayes, M.D.

"Women can benefit from a cardio rehabilitation program on many levels," says the cardiologist. "Unfortunately, it is grossly underutilized by women." Statistics show that women are 55 percent less likely than men to be referred to cardio rehab. Many who are referred are more reluctant to participate or drop out. Often, says Dr. Hayes, this is due to the pressure a woman feels, whether real or not, that she is needed at home in order for her family's life to return to normal.

Cardio rehab is an overall lifestyle program that offers prescriptive and monitored exercise tailored to the individual, education programs, and a supportive environment. It can also save your life, especially when you consider that hospital stays following a heart attack are shorter than they used to be. Research shows that rehab significantly reduces the risk of premature death or having a second heart attack.

If you have a heart attack and are not offered cardio rehab, ask for it, says Dr. Hayes. Then stick with it.

---

ing television. The point is, says Dr. Hayes, doing anything for any amount of time is better than doing nothing.

Tip 50: Go for Style

That is, your style. If you intend to stick with an exercise, it must be one you like. "If you can get out there and run, then great, but it isn't necessary," says Dr. Hayes. You may prefer biking, in-line skating, swimming, or just brisk walking. If it isn't a routine you enjoy, you are not going to stick with it.

Would you rather go it alone, join a group, or find a companion who will go along with you? If you do the buddy system, choose a person or group on a fitness and stamina level similar to yours. There is nothing more deflating than getting tuckered out when your exercise buddy is still pumped up.

Be realistic. Planning an exercise program that is too ambitious is a common mistake, says Dr. Hayes, because it is self-defeating. Even if you were a regular 5-mile runner 10 or even 5 years ago, but only walk now, you should not take off on a 2-mile-run tomorrow. You might be able to do it, but you'll regret it and become discouraged when you wake up the next day sore and with barely enough energy to get out and walk. If you want to begin running again, start by alternating walking with jogging for several minutes at a time. Gradually increase your running time. Remember, slow and steady is the rule.

Also, you may want to consider a new type of exercise rather than return to a program you had given up. The reason you gave it up is likely the reason you should not try it again. Set your heart on pleasure, not pain.

Give it time. As Dr. Hayes points out, exercise makes you feel good. Just give it time, especially if you are out of shape. Then stick with it. Even the most sedentary women will begin to feel the benefits after a week or two of regular exercise.

Don't give in to excuses. If you are ill or an obligation prevents you from exercising, just make sure you get back to it as soon as possible. It takes 6 to 8 months for an exercise regimen to stick. There are a lot of people who are addicted to exercise because of the great way it makes them feel afterward. It can even happen to you.

STEP RIGHT UP TO FITNESS

> "I now walk briskly every day and feel fortunate my heart disease was finally caught. I even walked down and back up the Rio Grande Gorge in New Mexico with no problems!"
> — Barbara, age 60

Let's say someone told you that you could perk up your mood, boost your energy, get physically motivated, shave a few inches off of your waist, and cut your risk of ever having a heart attack by 50 percent without ever stepping into a gym or putting on a pair of running shoes. You'd be all ears, right? Consider it said.

You can achieve all this and every other benefit already mentioned just by doing the easiest exercise there is: Walking.

Brisk walking is a no-excuses-allowed form of physical activity, says Dr. Hayes. It is easy, cheap, and enjoyable, factors that give it the lowest dropout rate of any form of exercise. No one leaves the women's heart center at Mayo Clinic without a free membership in the largest walking club in America—the 10,000 Steps Program. But it's a club anyone can join and all it costs is the price of a pedometer.

The 10,000 Steps Program is a federal government endeavor, sponsored by Shape Up America!, to help Americans improve their health through fitness. The goal of the program is to walk 10,000 steps a day. Only problem, say the people who invented the program, is that most people don't even come close to completing 10,000 steps a day. For most people, to get there requires at least 30 minutes a day of extra walking—the amount of time doctors say you need to do to get your heart in shape.

Tip 51: **Aim for 10K a Day**

Many women are convinced (or try to convince themselves) that they are active because they are busy running around all day keeping up with home, family, work, and whatever else obligates them away from joining a gym. Falling into bed dead tired at night is yet another sign that says life can handle no more. Quite possibly they are right—and there is an easy way to find out.

Get with the program. Slip a simple pedometer onto your waistband and let it track your steps through a normal day. If you're logging 10,000 steps a day then, yes indeed, you really are physically active. Congratulations! You'd make the U.S. Surgeon General (and envious others) proud.

The best investment you can make. There is no need to buy something fancy. For $30 or less, you can get a dependable, comfortable, and easy-to-secure pedometer with a built-in clock so you don't lose track of time. All you do is measure your stride, enter it into the gadget's memory, push a button, and off you go. It's a real motivator, says Dr. Hayes. And, those who have tried it will add, it is a challenge that is a whole lot of fun.

To figure out how many steps you typically take in a day, hook on the pedometer first thing in the morning and take it off just before you climb into bed. Do this for about three weekdays and also on the weekend. Write down your daily tallies and take the average.

You may want to average your weekdays and weekends separately if your routine varies greatly.

Prepare for the challenge. Let's assume that you have the necessary permissions to get started. Let's also assume your typical daily routine has you going about 3,000 paces, the high end for a typical sedentary woman. Experts recommend that you should increase your total of daily steps gradually. For example, set a goal of walking an extra 500 steps a day for two weeks. If you add another 500 steps every two weeks, you will have reached your goal in 28 weeks.

Keep account of your count. If you like the feeling of watching yourself succeed, keep a walking diary. Include anything you want: steps, distance covered, time, weather, your weight—whatever helps give you a sense of accomplishment. Keeping a diary is a good way to help you stay on track because you won't like looking at the blank spaces that remind you of days you missed! However, only keep a log if it is something you enjoy doing; otherwise it is a nuisance that may turn into an excuse to stop exercising.

Tip 52: **You'll Never Know It's Exercise**

Now you know: 10,000 steps is quite a feat! It puts you in motion for about 2-to-2½ hours a day. Even if you're chasing kids around, it sounds like a long haul. And if you have a desk job, it may seem next to impossible. But, really, it is not. Steps add up quickly. And finding ways to fit more in is a big part of the fun factor. Here are some ideas.

At work:

♥ Forget one-party interoffice e-mails. Deliver messages in person.

- ♥ Same goes for interoffice phone calls.

- ♥ Eat lunch somewhere within walking distance instead of driving distance.

- ♥ Take the stairs instead of the elevator (but only if it is safe to do so).

- ♥ Don't sit and think. Pace and think.

- ♥ Have one-on-one meetings in a walk-about, either around the hallways, around the building, or around the block.

- ♥ Don't hover outside your boss's office waiting for her to hang up the phone. Walk back to your office, then return. Repeat as many times as necessary.

- ♥ Keep your inbox in a spot that makes you get up and move to retrieve what's in it.

- ♥ Take the seat farthest from the entrance in meeting rooms.

- ♥ Put your outbox out of service and deliver your mail to the mailroom yourself.

- ♥ When someone stops by to talk, get up and walk around while you're chatting.

- ♥ If you haven't moved from your desk for a few hours, take a break and walk around the block. There are mental benefits in this, too!

- ♥ Don't sit for more than an hour for anything, including at meetings. Get up, walk to the back of the room, or excuse yourself on the pretense you need to make a call or use the restroom.

♥ Park as far from your workplace as is safely possible.

♥ Don't drive or take public transportation to work if you can walk.

At home:

♥ Hide the remote.

♥ When watching TV, do something active during the commercials—gather laundry, walk outside for some fresh air, check on the kids, take out the trash, make use of your hand weights, or walk circles around the sofa.

♥ Walk around while on the telephone.

♥ Walk the dog instead of letting him run in the yard.

♥ Unload the dishwasher and put back the dishes one plate at a time.

♥ Carry the groceries from the car into the house one bag at a time.

When out and about:

♥ Make one full circuit of the mall before you start shopping.

♥ Walk the escalators.

♥ Use the stairs instead of escalators and escalators instead of elevators.

♥ Don't jaywalk.

- ♥ Return your shopping cart back to the store.

- ♥ Do not use the drive-thru when doing your banking or dropping off dry cleaning.

- ♥ When you must drive to get somewhere, park at least a block from your destination.

Tip 53: Take a Midday Walk

On top of it all, you really do want to get some real exercise. A half-hour nonstop walk every day—about 2,000 steps—is all that is required to reach the minimum Dr. Hayes says will do your heart good. One study of older women found that those who walked briskly for 30 to 45 minutes just three times a week reduced their risk of getting a heart attack by 50 percent.

Just because it is walking, do not dismiss it as exercise. You're working your heart and muscles, meaning you should warm up and cool down just like a runner. This is what fitness experts say you should do:

Set your pace. Start out slowly for at least 5 minutes. This gives your muscles a chance to limber up, your body temperature a chance to warm up, and your blood flow a chance to increase gradually. Then, pick up your pace until you get to a comfortable speed. Check your pulse rate to find if you are in your target zone.

You don't need to walk hills to get exercise. Staying on level ground is fine. If you feel your walk isn't intense enough, try simply picking up the speed.

Cooling down is just as crucial as warming up and for the same reason. Make sure you end with a good 5 minutes of slow walking.

Before signing on at a health club, ask this question: Is the staff trained in CPR? "State-of-the-art" and "well-qualified" billings don't always translate to emergency situations. If the answer is no, it should be a deal breaker, especially if you already have heart disease. Heart patients should also inquire about the availability of an automatic external defibrillator and the location of the closest hospital emergency room. It is knowledge that will help make you feel more secure.

Posture is important. You should take long, smooth, heel-to-toe strides that feel natural. Keep your head up and spine straight but make sure you can see the road for possible obstacles. Keep your shoulders high and loose and let your arms hang loosely by your side. Use them to help power your walk as you start to feel fitness setting in. Breathe deeply.

Treat your feet right. If you need an excuse to buy a new pair of shoes, here it is. A good pair of walking shoes is the single most important piece of equipment. Second are socks that will wick away rather than absorb perspiration. Shopping for walking shoes can be a lot of fun because there are now so many different styles. Just make sure you buy for function over looks.

Shoes should support your feet, be firm at the heel, and have a flexible cushioned sole to absorb shock. The toe box at the front of the shoe should be roomy enough so you can wiggle your toes. Experts say leather is best but any breathable material will do.

This is a tip for shoe-lovers: If you walk at home and at work, then you will need two pairs of walking shoes. Having to cart exercise equipment around is a big hassle and having to remember to take walking shoes with you to work can be stressful. So, get an extra pair and keep them in a drawer in your office or work space.

THE FIT LIFE

> "I now do a lot of different types of exercise: walking, swimming, using a rowing machine, and lifting weights. Every once in a while, though, I need something new to keep me motivated. I've found medicine ball, yoga, pilates—I'm having a ball!" — Martha, age 70

Ask women who have succeeded and they will tell you that getting fit will change your whole life. Activity fills your blood with fresh oxygen, which is invigorating and makes you feel good all over. You'll have more energy to do more things, which means you'll be looking for new pursuits to use up your new-found energy.

Getting to the point where your fitness is something you want to do rather than something you have to do can take about 6 months. But there is no doubt about it; you'll know it when it happens.

Tip 54: Put Variety in Your New Life

One thing that can get in the way of reaching your fitness goal is

Walk briskly for a minimum of **30 minutes** every day.

monotony. Slavishly following the same regimen day after day can throw you off track on your way to fitness because it leads to boredom. Pursuing a variety of activities will prevent this from happening. For example, try alternating walking with bicycling or swimming. Play a game of tennis or take a low-impact aerobics class. Sign up for a pilates class or experiment with martial arts. Take scuba lessons.

Go to the MET. Scientists measure the intensity of an activity by the amount of metabolic energy the body requires to perform a task. The harder the intensity, the harder your heart works, the more calories you burn. In the end, how hard the activity is to perform—and your ability to perform it—depends on what kind of shape you are in. Based on these criteria, all activities, from sleeping to running a marathon, are given a rating based on what is known as a MET scale.

Scientists can use METs to calculate the average number of calories you can expect to burn during any activity. The activities listed in the following table were calculated by using METs. They are listed according to the type of workout, starting with the most intense. You can use it to figure out how hard you are working your heart, and roughly how many calories you'll burn. The numbers are based on a 125-pound woman doing the activity for 30 minutes.

ACTIVITY	CALORIES BURNED (PER 1/2 HR.)
Martial arts (karate, kickboxing, etc.)	285
Rope jumping, moderate	285
Running, 10-minute mile	285
Mountain biking	240

ACTIVITY	CALORIES BURNED (PER 1/2 HR.)
Running, 12-minute mile	230
Bicycling, moderate	225
Swimming laps, freestyle, moderate	225
Tennis, singles	225
Cross-country skiing	225
Snowshoeing	225
Beach volleyball	225
Snowmobiling	200
Tennis, doubles	200
Rollerblading	200
Racquetball	200
Backpacking	200
Ice skating	200
Snow skiing	200
Stream fishing	175
Water skiing	170
Scuba diving	170
Ballroom dancing	155
Working out in a gym	155
Playing outdoors with the kids	140
Ice skating	140
Aerobic dancing, low-impact	140
Stationary bicycling	140
Kayaking	140
Badminton	130
Golf	130

ACTIVITY	CALORIES BURNED (PER 1/2 HR.)
Carrying your clubs	155
Using a cart	100
Downhill skiing	120
Bicycling, 10 mph	115
Horseback riding	115
Yoga	115
T'ai chi	115
Water aerobics	115
Walking, 3 mph, flat surface	100
Walking, 2.5 mph, flat surface	85
Bowling	85
Volleyball, indoors	85
Billiards	70

Tip 55: Get with a Program

Here's the word some women just loathe: gym. Really, it only sounds intimidating. Gyms and health clubs are nice places filled with friendly people. Joining a gym is not your only option to achieve fitness, but today's health clubs offer a variety of fitness programs that can keep you from becoming bored.

If you feel clumsy or shy about not fitting it, that feeling will go away fast. You will get a lot of support from members and staff.

Meet resistance. The one important thing gyms and health clubs offer that you can't find anywhere else—unless you have a gym at work or home—is weight machines for resistance training. Ideally, says Dr. Hayes, you should combine you cardio workout with some resistance training a few times a week.

Working out with weights actually becomes more important as we get older. It strengthens and firms muscles and lubricates joints, which is especially important to women because it helps prevent bone loss and osteoporosis later in life. Stronger muscles improve stamina and balance. Also, muscle tissue is more metabolically active than fat, meaning you burn calories more efficiently all day.

You do not have to commit yourself to a year's membership at an expensive health club to try different things. Check and ask around. There are a lot of places and organizations that offer special-interest activities. Just do something!

7 Be **Weight** Wise

When it comes to protecting your heart, ignoring a weight problem is not an option. Here's why:

- ♥ The majority of women who have a heart attack are overweight.

- ♥ Women who are overweight, or more specifically, carry excess fat around the middle, have the highest lifetime risk of having a heart attack and dying from heart disease.

- ♥ Being overweight is a major contributor to high blood pressure, high cholesterol, and diabetes. In fact, 70 percent of women with diabetes carry around too much fat.

- ♥ Obesity is a leading contributor to metabolic syndrome, a cluster of risk factors that carries the dubious distinction of doubling your odds of dying from heart disease.

It is an unfortunate irony that for all the salads we eat, desserts we decline, meals we miss, and other obsessive efforts we make to lose a few pounds, American women are fatter than ever. More than half of us carry around extra fat that can lead to heart problems.

But here's the real irony. While American women are typecast as perpetual dieters who worship thinness, we are actually eating more than ever before. Statistics show that over a 30-year span, starting in 1971, the average calorie consumption among women has increased 22 percent—equivalent to an extra 335 calories a day. (In men, the increase is only 7 percent.) That means the average middle-aged woman is around 30 pounds heavier than she was in the early 1970s—coincidentally, about the same time that Dr. Atkins' high-protein diet hit the market for the first time.

It is certainly a troubling statistic, but it explains, at least in part, why obesity is increasing at an alarming rate. So, what are we doing wrong? Let's start with our devotion to a four-letter word: d-i-e-t.

A LIFESTYLE, NOT A DIET

"Why did I have a heart attack at 45? I had a significant family history, smoked, was overweight, and I didn't exercise. Like everyone else, I thought that being a woman ruled out any chance of having a heart attack. Boy, was I wrong!"
— Marcia, age 60

Somewhere along the way, the connotation of diet has changed from what Merriam-Webster defines as "food and drink regularly provided or consumed" to "deprivation of certain foods until a reduction in weight is achieved." And we attempt it again, and again, and again.

"From a health point of view, going on some fad diet temporarily is about the most unhealthy thing you can do to your body," says Dr. Robert J. Moore, a fitness and weight-loss specialist in Houston. "Dieting is self-defeating. The body is built to naturally protect itself from starvation. It's why dieting is so hard to accomplish and why 90 to 95 percent of people who lose weight gain most of it back."

What's so insidious is that our sacrificial efforts are paid back in pounds of extra fat that make their home in the soft tissue just under our skin. With every diet defeat, more fat calls your body home. Like other parts of the body, fatty tissue depends on oxygen and nutrients to survive. As fat accumulates, demand for these life-sustaining substances increases. This means the amount of blood traveling through the body increases. More blood moving through arteries means more pressure against the artery walls. And that's what sets you up for cardiovascular disease.

A women's heart study conducted at the University of Michigan in Ann Arbor demonstrated just how hard the cycle of gaining-losing-regaining, known as yo-yo dieting, can be on the heart. The long-term study found that women who yo-yo in weight five times within 1 year during their early and midlife years set themselves up for heart disease after menopause, even if they are thin at the time. They found that women who go through weight swings have lower than average blood flow to the heart.

Eating Heartfully

"Dieting through deprivation isn't natural," says Dr. Moore, who explains his food and fitness philosophy in his book, *Body of*

Knowledge. "What's natural is eating frequent, small meals of foods designed by Mother Nature. If it's processed, comes in a box, contains sugar or refined flour, it is going to threaten your ability to maintain or lose weight."

Tip 56: Ban the Ban on Carbohydrates

It's no coincidence that Mother Nature's food supply contains all of the foods that are known to be good for your heart. These foods— the fruits, vegetables, and grains that grow on vines, stalks, and trees—contain the essential vitamins and minerals we need to survive and provide us with carbohydrates, protein, and fat. "Most of nature's foods are low in fat and high in complex carbohydrates, the body's main source of fuel," says Dr. Moore. "It is just the way your body was designed to take in these nutrients."

Somewhere along the long, crowded road to slimness, we got sidetracked into believing that giving up carbohydrates was the shortcut to getting there. In truth, it's just another dead end. In fact, many health-care organizations such as the American Heart Association, American Institute for Cancer Research, National Consumers League, and the American Obesity Association have come down hard on low-carbohydrate diets, going as far as to say they are leading Americans down the road to poor health. Why? Because vegetables, fruits, whole grains, and beans—all carbohydrate foods—are linked to reducing the incidence of heart disease, stroke, diabetes, and many other diseases, such as cancer. In addition, high-fat, high-protein diets have been linked to causing the same problems.

A study conducted by Mayo Clinic set out to find the health

Atkins Not Female Friendly

Nearly half of American women are on some kind of diet on any given day, so it is likely at some time many, if not most, of us have tried a high-protein, low-carbohydrate program such as the Atkins' diet. How long did *you* last on it?

Anecdotal evidence has shown that men adapt easier and tolerate the diet longer than women. Now there is an explanation for it. It has to do with our biology.

Women have less serotonin, a natural hormone that controls the satiety center in the brain. Women manufacture only about half the serotonin that men do, according to researchers. When serotonin levels are up, we feel full. When levels are low, we get cravings and feel hungry.

Olga Raz, R.D., author of *The Bread for Life Diet*, found that a high-protein meal makes serotonin levels in the blood go down. "I have many women patients who complain that they can't stay on the Atkins diet, but their husbands do not have a problem with it," she says.

Bottom line: A diet that includes complex carbohydrates such as whole-grain bread is what works best for women.

risks, if any, for 29,000 older women who ate a relatively large amount of protein from red meat and dairy products, such as butter and cheese. They found that those who reported the highest intake of these foods had a 40 percent higher risk of dying from heart disease within the next 15 years than those who ate the fewest high-fat, high-protein foods. That was the conclusion even after researchers accounted for other dietary habits, plus exercise, smoking, and current weight.

"Carbohydrates don't make you fat," says Dr. Moore. "What makes you fat is eating the wrong kinds of carbohydrates; eating too much of anything, including carbohydrates, at one time; and eating too much overall."

Don't keep it simple. All carbohydrates, however, are not exonerated from prosecution in the fat wars. Carbs get their bad reputation from a specific sect called simple carbohydrates. They are easy to spot and easy to avoid because they are generally clad in white. White sugar and flours and all their spin-offs, especially sweets, baked goods, and white bread, are simple carbohydrate foods.

They are called simple because they are fast-acting, meaning that they rush into the blood system like bargain-hunters crashing through the doors at opening time on dollar day. This sends easygoing insulin and glucose (blood sugar) into a frenzy, causing them to rise and fall and rise again. The only way to stop the mayhem is to push the invaders out of the way—right into fat cells.

Complex carbohydrates work the opposite way. They are slow-acting, so when they enter the bloodstream, they don't upset insulin. The only time they are likely to cause trouble is if you eat too much. Complex carbs are easy to recognize because they are nature's foods.

Eat fruit one piece at a time. Vegetables, legumes, and grains are great sources of complex carbohydrates. Fruit is good, too, but you should be careful, says nutrition researcher Olga Raz, R.D., in her

To lose weight, reduce your intake of simple carbs—the whites—as much as possible and eat lots of **high-fiber complex carbohydrates**.

book *The Bread for Life Diet*. Fruit contains a sugar called fructose and, even though it is natural, too much at one time can upset insulin. She suggests eating fruit as your midday snack.

A simple secret. Of course, you can't go cold turkey on sweets. If you're going to eat simple carbs, do so early in the day and eat them with a little protein, suggests Dr. Moore. It will help regulate their absorption into the bloodstream. Keep sweets a treat by making them a rare indulgence.

Tip 57: **Lose Weight Naturally**

Mother Nature is a clever lady. The foods that are good for the heart are also good for the waistline. You will lose weight naturally if you focus your eating habits on the foods recommended in this book—that is, a diet low in saturated fat and high in complex carbohydrates. Get your protein from vegetables sources as much as possible, such as beans or soy products. Eat low-fat animal protein—more poultry (without the skin) than red meat, and only lean cuts of meat.

To lose weight, the American Heart Association recommends getting no more than 30 percent of your calories from fat. Make your fat preference the monounsaturated kind, like the fat found in olive oil and nuts. You can read about how to make monos part of a healthy diet beginning on page 71.

Eat a little a lot. Big meals have the same effect on insulin and fat storage as simple carbohydrates do, says Dr. Moore. In addition to making insulin work harder, they also make the heart work harder. When you eat, blood goes to the stomach to aid in the digestion process. A big meal requires a larger supply of blood, which means harder pumping action. That's why it's no surprise that many heart attacks occur following a big meal.

Many weight-loss experts, including Dr. Moore and Olga Raz, recommend eating as many as five or six small meals throughout the day. Smaller meals help your weight because insulin levels stay normal and fat storage is discouraged. This does not mean that you should eat more; rather you should eat less, but more often.

The Big Fat Felon

A clique of foreign substances known as trans fat has been charged with impersonating a natural fat and endangering the health of consumers by infiltrating our food supply. Though the evidence against it is strong, this oil-like substance, which has the peculiar ability to stay solid at room temperature, is still at large and invading the shelves of every supermarket and vending machine in America.

Based on the evidence gathered through scientific research, nutrition activists believe that arresting trans fat could prevent between 30,000 and 100,000 deaths a year from heart attack and help slow the rising obesity rate.

Trans fat, which has been at large for decades, was the brainchild of well-meaning manufacturers who wanted to ease the burden of feeding a family by doing part of the cooking and putting food in a well-sealed package until needed. The idea became an instant success and coined a new household term: *convenience food*. Trans fat was later adopted by fast-food restaurants because they could

To lose weight, **reduce your daily fat intake** to 30 percent of total calories or less.

Kids, Fat, and Heart Disease

If you need some incentive to lose weight, try this: Set an example for your children. Being overweight is not just a problem for adults. If obesity continues to grow at its current rate, scientists says, the lifespan of future generations is going to go down instead of up for the first time in history.

What's going to shorten their lives? Heart disease, for one. Obese children are already showing early signs of heart disease. One study of 343 extremely obese kids at Cincinnati Children's Hospital Medical Center found that they already showed signs of thickness of the heart. Their average age was 12.

The thicker the heart, the more likely the potential for reduced blood flow, which leads to a heart attack. Other studies are finding early signs of diabetes in children.

On the other hand, researchers at the University of Alabama and the Medical College of Georgia found that when obese children decrease body fat and increase cardio-vascular fitness, they reduce their risk for type 2 diabetes and heart disease.

make French fries crispier and sweets creamier. Plus, they could keep for months without spoiling.

Because trans fat is derived from vegetable oil, it was thought to be safer than saturated fat, a well-known hardened killer. But the process that turns it into trans fat (the oil is pumped full of hydrogen at high heat) didn't fool Mother Nature. She detected it as a foreign substance and blew the whistle on its harmful effects. Now trans fat is considered the most dangerous fat in our food supply, even worse than saturated fat.

Tip 58: Pass on the Trans Fat, Please

Unlike natural fats, which are both good and bad for you, trans fat can only mimic the bad side of fat. Like saturated fat, it clogs arteries. Unlike monounsaturated fat, which lowers bad cholesterol and raises good cholesterol, trans fat does just the opposite. That's bad. So bad, in fact, that the Food and Drug Administration (FDA) and the American Heart Association have declared there is "no safe level" for human consumption. Their best advice: Eat as little as possible.

Beware of fakes in disguise. Some manufacturers are putting out products that claim to be "trans-fat free." It is legal to make this claim as long as the trans fat content is under a half-gram per serving, not per package.

It is easy to figure out just how trans-fat free a package really is. Note the amount of total fat per serving on the nutrition label. Underneath the total grams is a breakdown of the individual types of fat and their gram content. Add up the grams of the individual fats. Say, for example, the total grams of fat per serving is 10. If the total of the individual kinds of fat listed comes to 8, then you can assume that those missing two grams of fat are trans fat. Eat two servings and you double your trans fat intake.

Other danger signs. Chemically, trans fat is known as partially hydrogenated oil. If you see these words or any phrases that contain the word "hydrogenated," or "partially hydrogenated," translate it to mean trans fat.

Palm's down. The image of palm leaves swaying in the breeze may make it sound innocent, but palm oil is a serious artery stuffer. Before trans fat was invented, palm oil was the common preservative used in packaged foods. It also made food taste good. But the nutrition enforcers came crashing down on palm oil because it is even worse than saturated fat.

Consumer watchdogs say that some manufacturers are retreating back to palm oil in an effort to keep taste appeal high until a substitute is found for trans fat. Palm oil, however, is also believed to be worse for you than trans fat. So, read the labels and keep away from palm oil.

Shop at health food stores. Manufacturers are spending millions to find a safer workhorse to replace trans fat, but are having a difficult time finding one that will make fast-food fries and packaged

---

Something Ventured, Something Gained

The United States is known as the land of opportunities, one being the opportunity to get fat. If a study of more than 32,000 United States immigrants is any indication, foreigners who move to this country can expect to grow with each passing year.

The research, conducted by Harvard Medical School, shows that after 15 years of living in the United States, immigrants have the identical susceptibility to gaining weight as the average Joe or Josephine. Unfortunately, it appears to put them at a greater disadvantage than their native-born neighbors when it comes to dealing with the repercussions. The same research found that only 14 percent had access to the proper health care that could help them correct the problem.

cookies and crackers taste the way consumers expect them to taste. Meanwhile, as the search goes on, trans fats are still at large.

You do not want to waste your fat allowance on oils that are not good for you, especially when you are trying to lose weight. Read labels when food shopping. Best yet, shop at health-conscious food stores. Places like Whole Foods Market and Wild Oats Natural Marketplace say they won't stock products containing trans fat.

Tip 59: Read Labels Suspiciously

The low-fat diet craze came to an abrupt end about a decade ago when manufacturers started feeding us low-fat and no-fat cookies, cakes, and crackers. They couldn't stock the shelves fast enough, and suddenly everybody was gaining weight on their low-fat diets!

Don't be misled by words such as *light* and *low fat* that you read on boxes and labels. They do not always tell the whole story. For one, there is the serving size. Even though serving sizes have been standardized by the federal government, some products still manage to post unrealistic sizes—such as a can of soup containing 2¼ servings. Twenty-ounce soft drinks are quite common nowadays, but to keep caloric content from being out of sight, the packager may list the contents as 2.5 servings at 110 calories per serving.

Then there is the fat content. Food guidelines tell us to think in terms of the percentage of calories we are eating each day from fat. Nutrition labelers apparently disagree because they list fat content by grams. To find out the percentage of calories from fat, you have to figure it out for yourself. Then there's 2 percent milk, which implies fat content. Or so you'd think. The two percent really refers to liquid weight, not the percentage of calories. Two percent milk actually translates to 34 percent of calories from fat; 1 percent is 23 percent of calories from fat.

Labels not only can be deceiving but they also can be wrong. In Florida, the FDA evaluated 67 diet products and found every single one was inaccurately labeled in some way. And this was not an isolated case. A test of popular protein and nutrition bars found 60 percent contained erroneous claims.

Tip 60: **Stay Out of the Fast-Food Lane**

Next time you're in such a mad rush that you only have time for a fast-food meal, slow down, take a big breath, and tell yourself that you deserve a break today. Take time to eat a real lunch. Fast-food restaurants are notorious hangouts for trans fat.

Nutrition experts rail that fast-food and chain restaurants with their super-sized portions and all-you-can-eat lures are a major contributor to the growth of the American waistline. And it is more than speculation. One study followed 3,000 women ages 18 to 30 for 15 years and monitored their fast-food habits. Those who frequented fast-food places two or more times a week gained an average of 10 pounds more than those who ate fast food once a week. They also had a two-fold greater increase in insulin resistance.

End of story.

LOSING WISDOM

> *"The first thing I did after my heart attack was work with a nutritionist, and then I changed my entire eating pattern. I joined the YMCA and suddenly became aware of my weight and body fat. Now, 19 months later, I have lost 64 pounds and 13 inches of body fat. And I eat well!"* — Barbara, age 66

If you are overweight, it is in your best interest to lose your excess pounds, especially if you've already been diagnosed with heart disease or have any of the major risk factors, cautions Sharonne N. Hayes, M.D., Director of the Women's Heart Clinic at Mayo Clinic in Rochester Minnesota. Being roughly 25 pounds overweight can lower good HDL cholesterol, raise bad LDL cholesterol, increase blood pressure, and induce diabetes. "Even a modest reduction in weight—5 to 10 percent—can reduce these risks," she says.

One study found that gaining 5 unneeded pounds lowered HDL levels by 2 percent in women (and 4 percent in men). In another study, losing 5 to 10 pounds lowered blood pressure enough for some women to go off their medication.

Eating Mindfully

You can ask just about any woman, and she'll say that she could stand to lose a few pounds. Remember, though, that Mother Nature didn't plan for all women to be model thin. Think of your weight in terms of your health. The surest way to find out if your weight puts your heart at risk is to find out where your weight falls on the body mass index (BMI) table on page 38. Shoot for a number on the lower side of 20. If you're between 25 and 29, you are considered overweight. A BMI of 30 or more is considered obese and puts you in the danger zone. Forty and over is considered morbidly obese.

If you have a BMI approaching the mid-30s or more, it likely means you have a lot of weight to lose. Dr. Hayes recommends that you see your doctor or a dietitian who specializes in weight loss for advice. A supervised program is your safest and best bet.

Tip 61: **Get Your Mind Set Right**

Women with a weight problem often have things other than hunger going on in their lives that contribute to overeating. Depression, chronic fatigue, marital problems, or money issues could contribute to the problem. Most times, though, women struggle with weight because of bad eating habits accumulated over the years.

"It takes considerable mental and physical energy to change your habits," says Dr. Hayes, "but you can do it if you are properly motivated." She suggests motivating yourself by focusing on the benefits of losing weight, such as more energy, better health, and the way you'll look and feel. Just don't ruin your motivation by setting unrealistic goals. Here are some suggestions from the Mayo Clinic:

Think process. Set your goals around process, such as eating only healthy foods and walking every day, rather than around outcomes, such as losing 10 pounds a month. Make sure your goals are measurable, like walking 30 minutes a day, but also make sure they are realistic.

Assess your eating behavior. Identify the situations that cause you to overeat. Do you eat when you are bored or anxious or home alone? Work out a plan to overcome them. Simply identifying them is not going to help you break the habit.

Enlist some support. In the end, only you can make the weight loss happen, but it helps to have support. Ask your spouse or a friend to encourage you and help you when you feel defeat coming on.

Sleeping Well?

Are you hungry when you're tired? Researchers think they know the reason. Lack of sleep can put your hunger hormones out of whack.

A study of 1,000 men and women found that those who slept poorly had increased levels of ghrelin, a hormone that increases feelings of hunger, and decreased levels of leptin, a hormone that helps suppress appetite.

The research, conducted jointly in the United States and England, defines poor sleep as less than 5 hours a night. But they concluded that less than 8 hours of rest a night can contribute to a weight problem.

Leave room for error. Expect setbacks and, most important, don't let them get you down. Just get right back on your program the next day or the next meal. Look ahead. Nothing is gained by chastising yourself for a mistake already committed.

Tip 62: **Eat a Little Less Each Day**

Be realistic, cautions Dr. Hayes. Healthy weight loss occurs slowly. Aim to lose no more than ½ pound to 1 pound a week. You can do this by eating 250 less calories a day than you are currently eating. For example, if you weigh 150 but you should weigh 135, it will take you about 4 months to lose 15 pounds. That's 10 percent of body weight, enough to achieve noticeable health benefits.

You can cut 250 calories a day just by making small adjustments in your eating habits. For example:

Cut your oil in half. Olive oil is great for your heart but it is still 100 percent fat. One tablespoon is about 120 calories. You shouldn't cut all oil out of your diet—it actually helps you to feel full—but you can cut back in ways that you will never notice it's missing:

- ♥ When a recipe calls for oil, cut the amount in half.

- ♥ Use sesame oil instead of olive oil in cooking. It contains very little saturated fat and the flavor is intense. A little goes a long way.

- ♥ Invest in a good nonstick sauté pan and use just enough oil to coat the pan when sautéing.

- ♥ Use low-calorie vinaigrette dressing on your salads. Olive oil-based salad dressings are a great way to get the benefits of monounsaturated oils, but if you want to lose weight, substitute flavored, vinegar-based dressings. You can make your own, but many bottled varieties are very tasty.

Make saving easy. Here are other ways to cut back on fat without missing out on taste:

- ♥ Reduce fat in baked goods by replacing half the butter with a combination of oil and milk. Or replace one-quarter of the fat with applesauce.

- ♥ Skim fat from sauces, soups, and gravies. The best way to do this is to let them cool, so the fat comes to the surface.

Raspberry Vinaigrette

Use a good quality raspberry vinegar.

2	tablespoons raspberry jam
6	tablespoons chicken stock
1	cup raspberry vinegar
1½	tablespoon olive oil
1	teaspoon Dijon-style mustard

Put the jam in a small bowl and whisk in the stock, vinegar, oil, and mustard. Keep in a sealed container and shake before use.

Makes about 1½ cups.

- ♥ Substitute two egg whites for one whole egg in recipes.

- ♥ Cut the fat in chocolate brownies by substituting prune puree for some of the fat.

- ♥ Use low-fat or nonfat yogurt to replace cream cheese, butter, or sour cream in recipes.

- ♥ Thicken soups and sauces with a puree of potatoes or instant potato flakes instead of cream.

- ♥ Use mustard, which has no fat and few calories, instead of ketchup and mayonnaise.

- ♥ Drink plenty of water every day, and avoid drinks that contain calories—except for your daily glass of wine. Caloric drinks do nothing to fill you up and they are full of sugar

- ♥ Start your meal with soup. Studies show that women who start a meal with soup naturally eat fewer calories throughout the day. Eat only broth-based soup; creamed soups contain too much fat.

- ♥ Leave something behind at every meal. It may not be what your mother taught you, but do it anyway. Leave behind a third of a 6-ounce burger on a bun, and you're halfway to success in your daily savings plan.

Tip 63: Practice Portion Control

Back in 1971, when the average woman was much lighter, so too were portions. It's estimated that portion size in restaurants and cookbooks are two to five times bigger than they used to be. That's not hard to believe; you can see it just about every time you go out to eat. Diners and family-style restaurants are notorious for their big servings.

This size guide comes courtesy of Mayo Clinic:

1   cup cereal = a fistful
½ cup pasta = an ice cream scoop
3   ounces meat = a deck of cards
3   ounces fish = a checkbook
1   ounce of cheese = four stacked dice
1   medium apple = a tennis ball
1   teaspoon butter = the tip of your thumb

HOW THIN WOMEN THINK

"I'm committed to learning more about my own heart condition and doing what it takes to stay healthy. I hope my life experience will help other women recognize and prevent their heart disease, because experience definitely is not the best way to learn!" — Jane, age 52

Yes, you could say some women were born to be thin. We all have friends who we could hate (if we didn't love them so much), because they can just eat and eat and eat, and not gain weight. If you are not one of them, you can blame it, at least to some degree, on your genes.

The propensity to gain weight is hereditary. If you are overweight, chances are around 40 percent that one or both of your parents have or had a weight problem. But even if you did inherit overweight genes, it is not a given that you will end up in oversize jeans.

Think back: How much of a family weight problem can be attributed to bad eating habits? Now, observe your naturally thin friends more closely. Chances are, they practice a lot of healthy lifestyle habits that contribute to their slenderness. French women are the perfect example.

Tip 64: Eat Like a French Woman

It's known as the French paradox. The French are obsessed with food, and their cuisine is the richest in the world. They eat bread and high-fat cheese and drink wine every day. Yet, French women don't get fat and they have a low rate of heart disease. That's because they:

- ♥ Eat fresh, seasonal foods. Processed foods aren't part of the French food universe.

- ♥ Don't snack between meals, unless it's a piece of fruit.

- ♥ Eat small meals. French portions are on average 25 percent smaller than portions in the United States.

- ♥ Avoid hard liquor.

- ♥ Walk everywhere.

- ♥ Love food and treat mealtime as an event.

It's obvious we'd love to be more like French women. Mireille Guiliano created a bestseller by revealing the secrets of staying thin with bread, wine, and even chocolate in her charming book, *French Women Don't Get Fat*. She sums it up quite nicely: "French women typically think about good things to eat. American women typically worry about bad things to eat." A few insights she reveals about French women include:

♥ They don't count calories or pounds. Their clothes are their scale.

Parmesan Crab Cake with Lobster Slaw

My decades-long search for the best crab cake ended at the Black Horse Tavern, a charming historic inn in Mendham, New Jersey. Chef Rocco Occhiato sautés the cakes, making a rich taste treat for calorie watchers.

Crab Cakes:

- 1 **egg, beaten**
- 2 **tablespoons Worchestershire sauce**
- 2 **tablespoons light mayonnaise**
- 1 **tablespoon fresh parsley**
- 4 **ounces grated fresh Parmesan cheese**
  Pinch black pepper
- 1 **cup breadcrumbs**
- 1 **pound jump lump crabmeat**
- 2 **tablespoons olive oil**

Lobster Slaw:

- 1 **head shredded green cabbage**

- They eat slowly and always sitting down.

- They eat small plates of a few courses, not one big plateful of different foods.

- They drink wine only as part of a meal, not as a cocktail.

- They love chocolate—the dark, bitter, heart-healthy kind—and eat it in small doses.

---

1 **whole carrot, shredded**
8 **ounces lobster meat, cooked and cut into chunks**
¼ **cup honey**
½ **tablespoon sugar**
½ **teaspoon salt**
   Pinch black pepper

To make the crab cakes, combine the first seven ingredients in a large bowl and mix well. Gently fold in the crabmeat. Divide and shape into 4 patties. Heat olive oil in a large frying pan and sauté at medium-high heat for about 5 minutes on each side, until golden.

To make the slaw, combine the cabbage, carrot, and lobster meat in a large bowl and mix well. In a separate bowl, combine the honey, sugar, salt and pepper. Mix well and stir into the slaw.

Divide the slaw among 4 plates and top with a crab cake. The slaw makes a tartar sauce unnecessary, but if you want a sauce, Chef Rocco suggests making a double batch of the slaw dressing and drizzling some over the top of the crab cakes.

Tip 65: Turn Off the Television

You know eating in front of the television is a bad habit. Now's there proof that it can make you fat. Every 2 hours you spend in front of the television increases the chance you'll end up obese. That's what doctors concluded after studying the leisure-time activities of 68,497 women who are part of the long-term, ongoing Nurses' Health Study. Specifically, they said, a TV habit increases your chances of ending up obese by 23 percent.

One of the reasons TV threatens your waistline is because many women are programmed to snack while watching television. A bad TV habit also implies a worse habit of avoiding exercise.

This doesn't mean you should never watch television. Just limit your viewing time. Using the same data, the researchers found that if women limited their TV viewing time to less than 10 hours a week, and walked briskly for 30 minutes or more every day, the rate of new obesity would go down 30 percent.

Tip 66: Eat a Healthy Breakfast

Thin women eat breakfast. They usually eat a healthy whole-grain cereal that keeps them content so they are not famished by lunchtime. Eating a healthy, high-fiber, whole-grain breakfast is especially important as we get older and our blood pressure and cholesterol get harder to control. Studies show that women over 65 who eat high-fiber or bran cereals and dark breads such as wheat, rye, and pumpernickel, have less heart disease than older women who eat refined cereals.

Tip 67: Don't Forget Your Daily Wine

Here's a study that perhaps, in part, explains the French paradox. It seems that drinking red wine may help stimulate a gene called SIRTI that can reduce the number and size of fat cells.

As diet expert Dr. Robert Moore explained earlier, when the body senses that it is getting fewer calories because you are dieting, it becomes more efficient at storing fat. Scientists found in animal studies that the SIRTI gene may have the ability to repress the protein that tells the body to store fat when food becomes scarce. It may also increase the burn rate of fat within cells. Also, in animal studies, researchers found that resveratrol, the key compound in wine believed to promote heart health, may even speed up the activity of this gene.

Tip 68: Get into Deficit Spending

At the end of the day, thin women are thin because they manage to burn up all the calories they take in. There are reasons why this

Exercise and Hunger

A study has now proven what women already know: Exercise makes us eat more. Though previous studies show that high-intensity exercise blunts a man's appetite, a study at the University of Ottowa found the opposite is true for women. The researchers found that women who exercised intensely ate more than women who exercised moderately and those who didn't exercise at all.

Bottom line? Exercise is worth doing, it is just not worth overdoing. Moderation rules.

happens. They have less fat, meaning they burn calories more efficiently. Fat burns calories slower than muscle does. Thin women generally have plenty of energy because they don't have extra weight to slow them down. And, of course, active people burn more calories than sedentary ones.

The number-one rule of weight control never changes. If you take in more calories than you expend, you are going to gain weight. Every 3,500 calories that sit unused inside your body turn into another pound of you. Conversely, to shed a pound, you have to burn an extra 3,500 calories. Exercise, particularly aerobic exercise, gobbles up calories, and continues to do so for hours after you stop, says Dr. Moore.

If you want to lose weight, you might have to step up your exercise goal. Thirty minutes a day is excellent for heart health and weight maintenance, but experts say that achieving weight loss primarily through exercise requires an hour a day. Depending on intensity, you can burn from 3½ to 7 calories a minute through exercise.

Swing your arms. Intense exercise, however, is not for the overweight and out of shape, warns Dr. Moore. But it is something you can work toward as you get thinner. Walk, stay active, and burn extra calories a little at a time. For example, carrying two-pound weights and swinging your arms while walking burns 5 percent more calories. Sitting burns more calories per hour than lying down, and standing burns more calories than sitting.

Do some mental arithmetic. Figure out how your average day plays out in terms of your activities and compare it to your food intake. Start walking more and increase your activity level gradually. Cut back on your eating gradually. Forget the fast food and the processed food. Instead, relax and enjoy a healthy meal of fresh foods. That's what thin women do.

8 Stress Happens

Anyone who doubts that men and women are wired differently should take a look at a group of married workers at a Volvo plant in Sweden. Researchers wanted to find out how stress affected men and women, so they hooked them up to all-day monitors that measured heart rate and blood pressure. When the men arrived home after a day's work, their blood pressures went down and their heart rates relaxed. But when the women walked through the front door, just the opposite happened!

The idea that stress is something only a man experiences was exposed as a fairy tale a long time ago, but medical doctors and psychologists acknowledge that there is still a lot to learn about stress and how it impacts the heart health of both men and women. They do know that stress provokes heart disease. They also know that stress affects men and women in very different ways. The Swedish Volvo workers are a classic example.

"To the men, arriving home at night was the end of the workday, the end of stress, a time to relax," explains Wayne M. Sotile, Ph.D., a leading cardiac psychologist and author of *Thriving with Heart Disease*. "For the women, walking through the front door only signaled the start of the second shift."

Add to it the fact that many men "just don't get it" puts female stress in a category all its own. "Women take a lot on themselves as the caregivers," says Dr. Sotile who, along with his wife, Mary, has spent the last 25 years helping men and women deal with the emotional fallout from having a heart attack. "Women by nature have the tendency to want to take care of others before themselves." A woman can walk around chronically stressed without realizing it. And that means she also does not know what it is doing to her heart.

A HOLD ON THE HEART

> *"I look back on that night in the ER and wonder why my classic symptoms were not taken more seriously. Yes, I was young; yes, I was female; yes I was in good health. That doesn't give anyone the right to dismiss my symptoms and deny that something was wrong."* — Cindy, age 30

Stress happens when something unexpected or unknown intrudes on your life. It could be anything from a sudden bang that makes you jump and your heart pound to the death of a close friend or relative that leaves you shattered and sad. When this happens, it sends your nervous system into action, blasting off protective hormones and brain chemicals like a rocketship launched into orbit.

In response, muscles tense, the heart starts to race, and blood pressure goes up. This increases the heart's need for oxygen. Small arteries also can constrict, which can put women whose arteries are already narrowed by plaque in peril.

The heart is built to withstand a certain amount of stress, but when stress is incessant—when you are tied in knots day after day after day—it creates a state of anxiety that can put your heart in jeopardy.

Stress is double trouble for women because of our biological makeup. When stress happens, the body releases a variety of stress-fighting hormones. That's good. But the turmoil also causes the female hormone estrogen to surge, then run for cover—and that's bad. Evidence shows that chronic stress reduces estrogen levels; and lower estrogen can lead to heart disease.

This was first observed in monkeys. A study at Wake Forest University Baptist Medical Center in Winston-Salem, for example, found that female monkeys, stressed due to their subordinate roles

Pressure On, Pressure Up

People who respond poorly to stress are likely to develop high blood pressure. In fact, the link is so strong that researchers can predict, among young people, who is likely to develop high blood pressure later in life simply by observing their reactions to stressful situations. One study of 4,000 people ages 18 to 30 found that those who get stressed out over things as seemingly harmless as playing a video game are most likely to develop high blood pressure by the time they reach 40.

in their group, became estrogen deficient. They also ended up with four times as much plaque in their arteries than the dominant female monkeys that maintained normal estrogen levels.

"We know from monkey studies that stress can lower estrogen levels to the point that health is affected, even though the animals still have menstrual periods," commented Jay Kaplan, Ph.D., one of the study leaders. To women, this suggests that an estrogen deficiency prior to menopause can predict a higher rate of heart disease after menopause.

STRESS, NOT STRAIN

> *"I had no experience with heart disease prior to a major 'unannounced' heart attack. I wasn't overweight, I didn't smoke, and I had low cholesterol and normal blood pressure. I was content with my life, employed in a job that I enjoyed, and newly engaged."* —Terry, age 51

For decades, the solution to stress was to avoid it, an attempt that Dr. Sotile sees as fruitless—and even stressful. "It was foolish to ever think that we can avoid stress. Stress happens. The problem isn't stress; it is the failure to recover from stress."

An example he likes to use is a dog darting onto the road as you are driving down the street. You slam on the brakes and narrowly avoid the animal. "The dog feels the stress of the situation, too, but by the time it gets to the other side, it can just lie down and go to sleep. But you behind the wheel will do any variety of things—yell, shake, cry, break into a sweat—anything but let the emotion go. You could even be rethinking it for hours. And every time you recall the event, you will have another stress reaction."

Stress that gets out of control and festers frays the nerves and stabs at the heart—what Dr. Sotile calls strain. "It is strain, not stress, that gets you." So, the idea is to be a little more like the dog and a lot less like the woman who almost ran over the dog. When stress happens, you might not be able to roll over and go to sleep, but you can learn to keep your cool.

How to Spill Relief

The flip side of the stress response is the relaxation response. "The only difference is that the stress response turns on automatically and the relaxation response doesn't. You have to trigger it yourself," says Dr. Sotile. Relaxation is good because it lowers your heart rate, slows your breathing, eases tense muscles, and even allows you to sleep more soundly.

Tip 69: **Take a Deep Breath**

When you feel tension starting to build, stop and take a deep breath. Inhale deeply through your nose, then exhale slowly through your mouth. Do it again. And again. This is good for the short-term and will lower your heart rate and make you relax, says Dr. Sotile. A more permanent technique is to breathe using your diaphragm, like newborn babies do. Most people breathe with their chest muscles.

Slow down your breathing. Diaphragmatic breathing, also known as belly breathing, is good because you take in more air per breath than you do breathing with only your chest. You don't have to inhale

> Learn to **manage stress**, not avoid it. Find the
> technique that works for you and practice it every day.

as frequently to get the oxygen you need. This means your breathing slows, your heart rate slows, and you relax. To learn the technique you will, at first, have to consciously pay attention to your breathing. Here's how you do it:

- ♥ To find your diaphragm, lie flat on the floor and place one hand on your stomach just below the rib cage.

- ♥ Inhale by expanding your stomach. If you are doing it properly you will feel your hand rise.

- ♥ Place your other hand on your chest. If you are doing it properly, this hand will hardly move at all.

This is really the natural way to breathe but most of us have to relearn it, says Dr. Sotile, and it can take some time. He says you can expect it to take a few weeks to master the technique.

Tip 70: Set Your Muscles Free

Many women are so used to tight muscles that the tension actually feels natural to them. This muscle-relaxing technique is recommended by Valerie Gennari Cooksley, R.N., a holistic nurse and author of *Healing Home Spa*. She recommends taking 10 minutes every day to set your muscles free.

Find a quiet spot with a comfortable place to lie down, such as your bed or sofa. Close your eyes and give yourself a minute or two to get calm and still. Focus your mind on your breathing and take deep, slow, and even breaths. Notice which parts of your body feel tense and which feel relaxed.

As you exhale, release the tension in your tight muscles. Start by concentrating on your feet. Inhale, then exhale as you ease and release the muscles in your toes, instep, then heel. Gradually move up your body until you reach the top of your head. When you are finished, remain quiet and relaxed for a few minutes longer.

As you do this on a daily basis, you should feel a shift from your body's tension; you'll gradually feel your body get looser and more supple, says Cooksley.

Tip 71: Just Close Your Eyes and Be...

...in a place you love to be. If you can daydream, then you can master the relaxation technique called visualization. Again, find yourself a comfortable place devoid of distractions. Sit or lie down and get totally comfortable.

Close your eyes and, through your mind's-eye, picture a place or scene that is special to you, such as a quiet morning beach. As you relax, let sound enter the picture—the call of the seagulls, the lap of the water against the shoreline. Hear the sounds, smell the sea air, feel the cool breeze wash over your face and brush through your hair. Continue the image as you feel a calm going through your body. Hold the image for as long as possible . . . and release.

Again, this may be a technique that takes time to master, but once you do, you can call on it anytime you find yourself short on patience, such as being stuck in traffic or waiting in long lines.

Tip 72: Close Your Eyes and Smell the Flowers

In addition to being a holistic nurse, Cooksley is a leading authority on aromatherapy, an alternative healing practice that uses concentrated botanical essential oils to achieve various psycho-emotional states. Recent research has found that smelling certain essential oils, or flower essences, can stimulate brain chemicals that control certain emotions. Rose, geranium, and lavender are among the essences that can help zap stress.

One drop is all you need. Essential oils are sold in small amber bottles that fit conveniently in a small purse. Whenever you are feeling stressed, just put a drop of oil on a tissue or handkerchief,

---

Buy Yourself Some Time

Studies show that women have an unrealistic image that the future will offer more free time than the present. We may feel overwhelmed about today, or even this week, but we see giant blocks of uncommitted time in the future. This is an illusion. As tomorrow turns into today and this week, we find we are just as busy.

The nature of time fools us, and we forget how many ordinary things can fill the day, explains Wayne Sotile, Ph.D. "If you're not careful, you'll end up with more and more things to do and less time to do them."

Try this experiment to find out how realistic you are about planning your time: Pick a 2-hour slot of time 2 weeks from now that is not committed to anyone or anything. Pencil it in to do nothing. Good luck!

---

put it close to your nose, and take several deep breaths. Inhale from the nose to a count of three and exhale through the nose to a count of six. In a sudden stressful situation, you can inhale straight from the bottle.

Only a drop or two is needed, says Cooksley. Essential oils are potent. For example, it would take 30 cups of herbal tea to get the same therapeutic effect as 1 drop of pure essential oil. Make sure to buy unadulterated oils or else you won't get the desired result.

Tip 73: **Concentrate on Nothing at All**

Meditation is a mind-body discipline in which you use your mind to reach a state that some practitioners describe as "wide awake, but not thinking." Meditation takes many forms, but the goal for all of them is the same: to free yourself of thought and put your mind and body in a state of total relaxation. It is a discipline that takes patience to learn, but most people who master it become lifelong disciples.

Studies have found that meditation can influence the body's health by bringing down blood pressure and eliminating physical signs of agitation. Studies focused on one form of the practice called Transcendental Meditation found that women are more successful than men at mastering the technique and also garner better results. Experts hypothesize this is because women are more committed to learning the practice.

Learning meditation takes training and practice. If it is something that interests you, your best approach is to find someone qualified to guide you through the experience.

Tip 74: **Slow Down!**

Driving with the steering wheel in one hand and a bagel in the other. Giving instructions to the babysitter while putting on your makeup. Working the phone while washing the dishes. Finishing your breakfast while walking out the door. You might call it multitasking, but Dr. Sotile calls it hurry sickness. It even sounds stressful!

"Multitasking may sound like a good idea, but it really is not good for your health," says Dr. Sotile. "So, slow down! It is the most effective way to get control over your life." When you slow down, you also calm down. Practice patience by practicing the following:

- ♥ Consciously walk, talk, and eat more slowly.

- ♥ Become a relaxed driver. Don't drive in the fast lane, and try to stay in the same lane. Avoid weaving in and out of traffic.

- ♥ Focus and think about one thing at a time.

- ♥ Start and complete one task before moving on to another.

- ♥ When you park the car, stay put for a few minutes and finish listening to the song or news broadcast that is playing on the radio.

- ♥ Take mini-breaks throughout the day to practice stress-release techniques.

- ♥ Establish calming daily rituals such as doing a crossword puzzle or reading for 15 minutes before bed.

- ♥ Don't interrupt others before they are finished talking.

💜 Tidy up after each task so clutter stays out of the way.
Mess causes stress.

"Life is, by its very nature, unfinished," reminds Dr. Sotile. "There is no use in hurrying."

TOXIC JOB SYNDROME

"I was dancing through life as a 46-year-old who looked like a 36-year-old. My job as a peace officer was tremendously stressful but also challenging and quite the status symbol. Then, as I was packing for a well-deserved vacation, the proverbial lightning bolt struck and changed my life forever. I had a heart attack." — Penny

Many men, and even some women, believe that stress did not become a "woman's problem" until women put on trousers and started to climb the corporate success ladder. But that is not the case at all.

Studies show that men and women in power positions suffer the lowest risk of stress-induced heart attack. And that goes for women who are married or unmarried, with kids or without. The kind of job stress that leads to a heart attack is most often caused by being in a high-demand job without authority or decision-making power—a profile more common to women than men. As we know, life at the top is still largely a man's domain. In fact, the worker least likely to be affected by heart-related stress is a high-ranking executive male with lots of authority and a high salary.

Then there is job number two, the "second shift" of tending to home and kids, the kind of stress that mothers know best. Working moms can find themselves in a stress cycle—kids, career, home—each with its own set of energy-draining demands. It leaves them

---

Bliss at Work

Clear the air of stress with this aromatherapy mist recipe developed by Valerie Gennari Cooksley, R.N., who bottles her own blends at Flora Medica, her small company near Seattle, Washington. This blend was designed to lift your spirits and relieve job tension. She suggests spraying it in your office the first thing after you arrive at work.

All the oils recommended in this blend contain stress-releasing properties. Keep it in a drawer in your work space. The aromas are strong, so only a small squirt is necessary.

Blissful Office Blend

8 drops lavender oil

2 drops lemon oil

2 drops bergamot oil

1 drops geranium oil

4 ounces water

Combine the oils in a clean, glass mister with a light spray nozzle. Add the water. Shake well before each use.

strung out, overworked, short on time, and habitually tired. And who's to blame? Well, actually we are.

A recent study showed that when given the option, a working woman will willingly volunteer to take on the additional duties of a full-time, stay-at-home mother. Yes, superwoman is indeed alive, well, and stressed out. As Dr. Sotile points out earlier in this chapter, we are biologically programmed to be all things to all people—the nurturer, the perpetual caregiver. While it may be an instinct that we can't shed, there are ways we can make life a whole lot easier on ourselves and, as a result, a whole lot happier and healthier.

There are companies that accommodate wage-earning couples and single moms with options such as job sharing, flexible hours, and at-home work stations. Unfortunately, a lot of women are not in positions that qualify for these perks. "Most women have jobs where they have to be at work from 9 to 5, and sometimes even longer to meet a deadline," says Filomena Warihay, Ph.D., founder and president of Take Charge Consultants near Philadelphia.

Where's the Balance?

"Working women, and working mothers especially, are always being told that they need to put balance in their lives, and when they can't do it, it only makes them feel even more stressed," says Dr. Warihay, who, as a corporate consultant and leadership trainer, has counseled thousands of working women. "It is foolish to think that you can be well-balanced between work and home all the time. It isn't like that in real life."

Tip 75: **Let Balance Find You**

Accept the fact that there are days when your home life takes priority and days when your work life takes priority, says Dr. Warihay. Some days you might have to work late to get a report out or to help the boss, and that means your family has to do without you. Some days, when a child is sick or there is a school event, then your home life should be the priority. "Trying to find balance only makes you unbalanced," she says. "If you just let life happen, balance will find itself."

This is the philosophy she has been following since she joined the work force as a secretary nearly 40 years ago. Focusing only on what is important at the moment is what helped her work full-time, raise four children, take care of the house, and go to school at night.

Tip 76: **Take Care of Priorities Only**

Put the most important things you must do at the top of your list—always. "Don't worry what is on the bottom," says Dr. Warihay. "Just take care of the important stuff. Something doesn't become a priority just because it's been sitting there longer than everything else."

If there is routine work that you just hate to do, find a way that you don't have to do it. If you can delegate, then do so. If you can't, explain to your boss why it is in his, yours, and the company's best interest that it is better done another way. Just make sure you have the solution, says Dr. Warihay. Otherwise, you become the problem instead of the problem-solver.

Tip 77: Get Out of the Office Every Day

Mandatory breaks are required by law for a reason. Take at least a 30-minute break away from the office every day, says Dr. Warihay. It is a rule she has followed her entire work life, and it sure hasn't hurt her career.

"When I first started out, I would bring a bicycle to work, store it in the basement, put on a pair of shorts at lunchtime, and go for a half-hour bike ride," says Dr. Warihay. "Back then, it was unheard of. One of the other secretaries told me I was going to get in trouble. I said, 'So go and report me. I'll go along with you.' "

Tip 78: Don't Obsess Over a Messy Desk

Take a look around tonight on your way home. How many offices do you see where the desk is clean and clear of work?

"If you see one, then it's the desk of someone who's been fired," jokes Dr. Warihay. But she is only half kidding. "People who have clean desks all the time are sending the message that they don't have enough work to do and that they are not needed. I always tell people never to leave work at night with everything finished. When it is time to go home, go home!"

Whatever you don't finish today can get done tomorrow. Look at it this way, she counsels: If your job is such that you can't get away for a half-hour, either you are doing something wrong, or you should find yourself another job.

9 Don't Worry, Be **Happy**

How fitting that the icon for love is the heart. It symbolizes our emotions at every level, from the flutter of a promising new relationship (at any age!) to the heartbreak of broken dreams.

The impact of emotions on our heart health is difficult to quantify, doctors say, because feelings are as individual as fingerprints. But researchers are convinced that mental health is just as important as physical health when it comes to protecting the heart, especially for women. Why? Because women by nature are emotional—more emotional than men. The proof is found in the way we respond to stress, says Wayne M. Sotile, Ph.D., a pioneer in the practice and study of cardiac psychology.

It has long been known that the moment when stress strikes, the body starts to pump various hormones to help us deal with the situation. Men get a surge of adrenaline, the "fight-or-flight" hormone that also can give them the super-strength to lift a car off of a child's injured leg.

Women secrete adrenalin too, but they mainly secrete oxytocin, known as the snuggle hormone because it is the same hormone women secrete when breastfeeding.

Oxytocin is what gives us the "tending instinct," explains Dr. Sotile, the author of *Thriving With Heart Disease*. "Rather than fight or flee, as men are prone to do, a woman's inclination is to tend or befriend. It's the reason why when something upsetting occurs, a man wants to withdraw and a woman wants to talk about it." It is also the reason why stress can be particularly hard on women. Mismanaged stress enveloped in emotions can spiral into unhappiness and negative feelings.

There is plenty of evidence to link emotional negatives such as anxiety, worry, depression, bad moods, hostility, loneliness, and even a bad marriage to an increased risk of a heart attack or dying early from heart disease. For example, a review of seven studies that tracked the emotional health of more than 36,000 men and women found that those who had been diagnosed with clinical depression were twice as likely to develop heart disease as those who just experienced occasional depressed moods. And the clinically depressed were three times as likely to develop heart disease as those who reported no depression. This was true even for the clinically depressed who otherwise were considered in good health.

Other studies show that people who become depressed after having a heart attack heighten their risk of having another one within the following 18 months.

Now, here is why this is important information for you:

- Women are twice as likely as men to suffer from all forms of depression and twice as likely to die from untreated depression.

- Fifty percent of women recovering from a heart attack experience some form of depression or anxiety.

- Woman who lack strong personal relationships are 2½ times more likely to die early from heart disease than women in the same state of health who have a strong, satisfying social network.

- Women who are in mutual loving relationships are least likely of all women to end up with heart disease.

- Chronic worriers are two to four times more likely to have a heart attack than women who are able to stay calm in the same situations.

- Women who display anger and hostility have been found to have high levels of C-reactive protein, a sign of internal inflammation that is believed to aggravate the hardening of the arteries that leads to a heart attack.

WHY SO WAN?

"There is no way for me to describe the fear and anger I felt from having a heart attack. I suffered from physical and emotional pain, terror with every flutter of my heart, and tremendous anger that such a thing could matter to me."
— Maria, who had a heart attack at age 54

Researchers are unclear as to why depression can set you up for a heart attack, but doctors have observed a correlation between the two. Women who are depressed show signs of rapid heart rate, high blood pressure, and elevated cholesterol. Depressed people also have been found to have abnormal blood platelet activity, making it easier for clots to develop in the arteries and cause a heart attack.

Depression also upsets the body's hormonal balance. "Depression prompts the brain to release stress hormones that can cause heart rhythm disturbances or arrhythmias—the kind that can lead to sudden cardiac death," says Dr. Sotile. "Meanwhile, the brain releases fewer calming hormones, which aggravates stress. For women recovering from a heart attack, it decreases the chances of a full recovery."

On the flip side, a positive attitude offers huge rewards—among them the ability to ease tension and anxiety and head off a heart attack. "The happiest and healthiest people aren't blessed with extraordinary good fortune," counsels Dr. Sotile, "but they do devote more energy to basking in life's pleasures than they do to clenching their teeth over its letdowns."

Changes in Attitude

Just how bad can a bad attitude be? Really bad. When it comes to endangering a woman's heart, research indicates that anger and its explosive fallout rank as high as and possibility even higher than smoking. "For a woman with heart disease, a fit of anger more than doubles her risk of having a heart attack over the next 2 hours," says Dr. Sotile.

How Anger Explodes

When you feel rage burning, your body is going through other reactions that you can't feel, and this is where trouble brews. When you overreact, so do your stress hormones, causing fat levels in the blood to shoot up. "It heightens your physical reactions across the board," says Wayne M. Sotile, Ph.D. "The flow of hormones slows the removal of fat from the blood and crowds it with a surplus of red cells."

This process is called sludging and it can block off hundreds of tiny blood vessels for as long as 12 hours. This is why researchers warn that eating a high-fat meal when you are angry can trigger a heart attack.

Though most studies on hostility have been conducted on men, research shows there are consequences for women with hot tempers. One 4-year study conducted at the University of California San Francisco Mount Zion Women's Health Clinical Research Center monitored 800 menopause-age women with known heart disease for signs of hostility. Hostility was defined as signs of cynicism, anger, mistrust, and aggression. Researchers found that the women who showed the most signs of hostility were twice as likely to have a heart attack or die from heart-related problems than their more mild-tempered peers.

This does not mean anger is a risk only for older women. In fact, researchers analyzed the risk factors of 500 men and women under the age of 50 who had been hospitalized for a heart attack. All of them scored higher than average for signs of hostility.

Tip 79: **Keep a Cool Head**

Do you think venting your anger in ear-piercing decibels is the way to go? It's a belief as irrational as anger itself. Most women tend to hold their anger in, but that isn't good, either. Both extremes are equally risky and affect the wiring of your heart in a negative way. For a woman who has had a heart attack, either one can be lethal.

So, what are you supposed to do? Take the middle ground. Or, as Dr. Sotile puts it, "You need to learn to be appropriately assertive." For women who keep anger locked inside, the solution is straightforward, but not necessarily simple. Let your feelings be known, but not in a way that will inflame the situation.

For people prone to angry outbursts, experts offer these tips:

Keep a hostility log. This might sound trite, but people are often so busy being angry that they don't pay attention to what is pushing their buttons. "Other people may turn up your thermostat, but it is your anger," he says, "and you must learn to take responsibility for it." People often tend to fire their anger in the wrong direction. For instance, let's say you let the desk clerk really have it for losing your hotel reservation, though the real reason you are so angry is because you are running behind schedule and will be late for an appointment. The point: You need to identify your anger triggers and patterns.

Count to 10—or even 100—if necessary. It works! Dr. Sotile likes to quote author Ambrose Bierce when discussing the consequences of an angry outburst: "Speak when you are angry, and you will make the best speech you will ever regret."

Sleep on it. "If you have an anger habit, it means your calming response isn't kicking in on its own, and you must deliberately calm yourself down," says Dr. Sotile. Give yourself time to rationalize the situation that is making you so angry. Exercise has been shown to be an effective antidote for anger. So have the relaxation techniques recommended in Chapter 8. Sometimes it is just a good idea to sleep on it and see how you feel about the problem in the morning.

Assert yourself appropriately. If you've given yourself time to work through what happened and you are still upset, then it is time to assert yourself. Here's what to do:

- ♥ Don't swear, insult, or accuse.

- ♥ Separate the person from the problem. It is the situation that is upsetting you, not the person you feel created the problem. Getting personal, at best, hurts feelings and, at worst, destroys relationships.

- ♥ Use "I" statements that express how you feel instead of "you" statements that express what another person is doing to you.

- ♥ Offer an appropriate solution.

- ♥ Smile and say, "Thank you for listening."

Tip 80: Let Go of the Grudge

Holding a grudge is hard on your heart because it creates personal stress equal to that of a major event, such as a death in the family. It is also bad for your psyche because the low-grade anger numbs you into self-pity and unhappiness.

Studies show that learning to forgive, even something as hurtful as betrayal by a friend or spouse, has both physical and emotional rewards. One study found that forgiveness can help improve blood pressure and other stresses on the heart.

Easier said then done? Not really, says Dr. Sotile, once you realize that the biggest beneficiary of forgiveness is yourself. "Realize that forgiving is not condoning and it is not forgetting. It is also a powerful display of maturity."

Use these words. *I am forgiving you for my sake.* It will give you an overwhelming feeling of relief, says Dr. Sotile. "There is no grudge in the world worth dying over."

The other thing to do, he says, is to talk it out. "Let the person know how much he hurt you and how you feel. Tell him that you are doing this for yourself and not for him." Just don't harbor unrealistic expectations, he warns. "Don't expect the other person to change."

Tip 81: **Take the Cure for Worry Sickness**

It's Friday night and you're up late biting your nails and staring at reruns on TV. Your stomach is in a giant knot over the thought that your daughter may or may not be home safe and asleep in her bed— even though it is impossible to know because she is 2,000 miles away at college.

The phrase "worried sick" is very apropos when it comes to worry warriors. Chronic worriers, says Dr. Sotile, "literally take their anxiety to heart." Studies show that women who worry all the time are two to four times more likely to have a heart attack than women who know how to stay calm.

Worry is just an out-of-control form of pessimism. It's a sign that you've developed a negative thinking habit to the point where it has taken over your imagination. Just like any bad habit, you can learn to get over it.

Schedule worst-case scenario time. Taking the cure involves a daily exercise in which you contemplate irrational thinking while your mind is still rational. Once you're in the throes of a worry binge, it is difficult to get a grip on reality. So, schedule worry time

---

Sip Your Worries Away

As the mother of two college-age twin sons, aromatherapist and holistic nurse Valerie Gennari Cooksley, R.N., knows the meaning of the word "worry." She also knows how to avoid it: "Relax and stay busy doing things you enjoy," she advises.

She also relaxes by sipping cups of this homemade brew made with calming herbs and flowers.

No Worries Herbal Tea

- **2 parts chamomile flowers**
- **2 parts lemon balm herb**
- **1 part catnip herb**
- **1 part lavender flowers**
- **1 part peppermint leaves**
- **1 part rose petals**
  Pinch of fresh ground nutmeg

Combine all the ingredients. Keep the compound in a tightly sealed container in the pantry. When you are ready for tea, steep 2 teaspoons in a cup of hot water for 5 minutes and strain. Then sit back and drink your worries away.

---

every day. Dr. Sotile suggests doing it early in the day, before your mind has the time to crank up the worry alert. Then, get a pencil and paper and answer these questions:

- ♥ What do I worry about?
- ♥ What am I worried will happen?
- ♥ What is the worst thing that could happen?
- ♥ What will I do if it happens?

Your rational mind will see that you are creating fantasies and fantasizing catastrophes. When you are able to see them rationally, you will see how illogical they are. Worry is stress, but stress of your own creation. It happens because you don't manage it. The relaxation techniques suggested in Chapter 8 can be just as useful to banish worry as they are to reduce stress.

Fill your mind with happy thoughts. Idle minds breed worry sickness. When you are occupied doing something enjoyable, you don't have time to work yourself into a frazzle. If a "worry" event is coming up, plan to do something you thoroughly enjoy and preferably with someone who can help keep you distracted.

If worry interferes with your life to the point that it makes you unhappy or depressed, you should consider seeing a counselor.

Tip 82: Get Rid of Toxic Friends

Every workplace, neighborhood, and extended family has them—cynical and sour-natured people who see rain where everyone else sees a rainbow. They love pulling others under their clouds. Don't let them do it to you!

Toxic people come in various shades of black but they all share something in common: They can kill a sunny mood just by showing up in your doorway. Our natural instinct to nurture makes many women suckers for these types of people. Is this really how you want to spend your energy?

Don't let toxic friends pull you into their sphere of negativity. Life is stressful enough. Don't make it worse by associating with people who make you angry, upset, or depressed. This advice is particularly relevant to women who are recovering from a heart attack. "Choose wisely how to spend your precious life's energy," Says Dr. Sotile.

LAUGHTER IS GOOD MEDICINE

"My heart attack 2 years ago actually saved my life in the proverbial sense. I'm much happier, doing the things I like and living my life the way I want. I feel less stress and am enjoying things in a renewed way." — Cindee, age 34

When was the last time you had a good belly laugh? If you can't remember, then you are probably taking life, and yourself, much too seriously.

A daily dose of laughter is right up there with wine and chocolate when it comes to pleasures that can do the heart good. When researchers at the University of Maryland Medical Center in Baltimore tested the humor quotient of 300 men and women, they found that those with heart disease seemed to lack a funny bone.

While some people can laugh at themselves for silly foibles such as locking themselves out of the house in their night clothes, those with heart disease fail to see the humor in it. People with heart disease, says researcher Michael Miller, M.D., are just more uptight. The researchers found that people with heart disease were 40 percent less likely to see the humor in a variety of events others think of as quite funny.

The idea that a sense of humor is important to your health may sound, well, laughable, but it really should be taken seriously. Laughter is good for the heart in many ways. For one, it is an automatic stress-buster. Research at the University of California at Irvine found that just anticipating a funny event can decrease levels of stress-causing chemicals and increase levels of tension-releasing chemicals. Laughter also causes the tissues that form the lining of blood vessels to expand, thereby increasing blood flow. One study found that a good time that includes a lot of laughter can have the same healthful effect on blood flow as an aerobic workout.

Laughter is not something you want to take lightly. If it takes a lot to tickle your funny bone, here's what to do.

Tip 83: Laugh a Little Every Day

Take a look in the mirror during the day and study your expression. Keep in mind that what you see is what others see. It is hard to imagine the lighter side of life if you are staring at a tense face.

Laughter melts tension and that helps to lift your spirits, lighten your expression, and give you a better feeling of self-worth. "Laughter

Laugh every day. It's good for your heart and your emotional health.

is good medicine," says Dr. Sotile. "It is also contagious."

If you are around people who are laughing, you will be laughing, too. Or, at least you should be. If not, you need to ease the tension in your life. Here are a few ways to practice.

Laugh at yourself. Try laughing at yourself instead of getting angry when you do something stupid. Admit your faults instead of trying to cover them up. It will help you maintain perspective.

Laugh with others. Even if it is at your own expense! They may be laughing at you, but only because it really is funny. It's important that you, too, understand the humor in what you did.

Practice smiling. Consciously put a smile on your face and acknowledge at least three people you don't typically interact with each day. "When you smile at others, they will smile back," says Dr. Sotile. "It will make you both feel good."

Tip 84: **Watch Funny Movies**

Why cry when you could be laughing? In fact, research shows that watching a funny movie is therapeutic. Researchers at the University of Maryland proved this when they measured blood flow to the hearts of a small group of heart-healthy young men and women as they watched a 15-minute segment of the comedy movie *Kingpin*. Blood flow increased an average of 22 percent, comparable, they said, to the increase brought on by running or riding a bicycle.

Two nights later, the same group watched 15 minutes of the gut-wrenching World War II movie *Saving Private Ryan*. It had the opposite effects. Blood flow decreased 35 percent.

Laughing, concluded the researchers, can be one way to help prevent heart disease.

PEOPLE WHO NEED PEOPLE

"After my heart attack, I felt so alone and isolated. One day, I found myself wishing that I was an alcoholic so I could go to AA and have someone to talk to." — Judy, age 40

It is no surprise that being happily married ranks high on the happiness chain, but there is actually scientific evidence that shows it is good for the heart in more ways than one.

Researchers at San Diego State University tracked the health and happiness of 493 women for 13 years and found a correlation between the state of their marriages and the state of their hearts. Women who reported close and loving relationships with their husbands were less likely to have weight, cholesterol, and blood pressure problems. They also reported feeling less stress and depression than women in less-satisfying or troubled marriages.

Studies also show that men and women in long-term intimate relationships who have had heart attacks have a much lower death rate 5 years later than those who don't share a close bond with another person.

On the other hand, a bad relationship causes more trouble for women than it does for men who have had heart attacks, research from Sweden says. For a woman, it is marital stress, not work stress, that is the better predictor of whether she will have another heart attack.

What it all boils down to is that love matters. "The companionship of someone who cares about you—someone in whom you can confide your deepest thoughts, fears, and hopes—will not only enrich your life but could actually save it," says Dr. Sotile.

Happy Marriage, Healing Heart

Marital stress is toxic.

"A bad marriage can contribute to a heart attack and a healthy marriage contributes to heart health," says Dr. Sotile. Sadly, the majority of women in an unhappy marriage will quietly endure and just hang in there. But it still frays at the edges of her heart, both emotionally and physically.

It is much more common for the husband to find outside interests to fill the void simply because a man has more opportunity Men are generally not saddled with the responsibilities of house and home. Even women who do have friends and outside interests find they don't quite fill the void of unhappiness at home. Dr. Sotile counsels couples with troubled marriages and has seen many happy outcomes. "Marriages that go bad don't have to stay bad," he says.

Happy marriages often turn into unhappy marriages because husband and wife start out believing that they are so happy and in love that they won't have to work at staying that way, he explains. No couple is that lucky. Marriage, he says, is always a work in progress.

Tip 85: **Give Love to Get Love**

The traits the San Diego researchers used to gauge marital bliss were togetherness, mutual interests, open communication, and the two key things most often reported missing from a happy marriage: great

---

How Great Was That!

Wild and crazy sex won't cause a heart attack any more than passive and boring sex. In fact, the chances that any sex will cause an attack in him or you is one in 2.5 million. If you've already had a heart attack, you're chances are only slightly higher.

"Fearing sexual activity is very normal after a heart attack," says Wayne Sotile, Ph.D., who helps couples get over the emotional obstacles after one of them has had a heart attack. "You will have sex again. When your doctors says it's okay, it's okay."

He pooh-poohs the idea that getting too hot and heavy is dangerous: "Far more perilous than making love on the couch is sitting on the couch for hours and watching TV."

---

sex and financial compatibility.

Whether you want to keep the bliss in your relationship or are looking for ways to get it, here is what marriage therapists say are the hallmarks of a good marriage:

Communicate openly, often, and with kindness. "If you want to cultivate and maintain intimacy, you must communicate," says Dr. Sotile. Communication must be involved in every level of your relationship, including sex. Communication that is accusatory and negative will erode a relationship. It's just a form of hostility. Examples are put-down statements that lead with: "You never..." or "Why can't you..." or "Why don't you ...."

You probably think about him every day, right? Tell him "I was thinking a lot about you today." Say "I love you." Why just think it?

Other things Dr. Sotile suggests.

- ♥ Listen, even if what you are being told is not that interesting or important to you. Convey that you are listening with nods and assents.

- ♥ If you can't agree on an issue, agree to respect your differences.

- ♥ Remind rather than nag; suggest rather than complain.

Spend time together. Sure, this means getting a babysitter, if necessary, and going out by yourselves, but it also means sharing your lives in other respects, such as household duties. Your husband might be more open to cleaning the house together instead of taking turns. Take walks together, meet each other for lunch, read the same book at the same time and discuss it. Talk about your love life and ways to refresh it.

Get a little help. Keeping a marriage happy takes effort, and resolving a bad one takes more effort. It is not always easy, or even possible, to work through your troubles by yourselves. For some couples, a marriage counselor might be the answer.

The Gender Gap

By nature, women crave an emotional connection to others—we are the ties that bind. Not so for men. The reason has to do with our biological chemistry. As explained earlier, men secrete the hormone that gives them the natural instinct of fight and flight. A woman's natural instinct is to tend and befriend. We care. We nurture. We want friends and we want to be a friend.

The force of this yearning became blatantly clear when researchers found that a lack of social support can damage a woman's health. For example, one study of more than 500 heart-attack patients showed that women with few close relationships had a slower and tougher recovery than men. In fact, the lack of a social network did not appear to affect the mens' recovery at all.

The researchers, from Ohio State University, concluded that "friendship and companionship are extremely important for the health and well-being of women." They are so important, it appears, that their absence can even contribute to heart disease and increase a woman's chance of dying from a heart attack.

Researchers at the University of Florida College of Medicine in Tallahassee focused on the health of 503 older women with angina (chest pain initiated by exertion or stress) and found that those who had the fewest friends were at risk for dying younger than women who had a lot of friends. This was true whether they were married or unmarried. The only difference in their health was that women with few friends also felt emotionally distressed.

Tip 86: Create a Caring Social Network

Friendships are so important in a woman's life that one survey of more than 300 women, average age 59, associated quality of life with having a supportive social network.

The Florida research indicates that the larger the social network, the better for your heart. A network of six or more friends appeared to have the best influence on health. "Being married helps and having one or two close friends is even better," reported the researchers. "The more support, though, the better."

Be a joiner. There is nothing complicated about having a social network. Friendships develop at work, in exercise groups, and at church. So, make the effort. Having friends who care will make life seem a whole lot better.

Tip 87: Offer a Little Help to Your Friends

As traditional caregivers, more than half of American women will at some time in their lives take care of a sick, disabled, or dying family member. What is hardest on her—and, unfortunately her health—is caring for an ill spouse. In fact, she may even experience more emotional stress than her sick husband.

One study of male heart-attack survivors found that their wives had higher levels of depression and anxiety than they did. One reason is because the wife is there to support her husband's feelings, but there is no one to help support her.

"Women tend to take on these duties without giving up duties in other areas of their lives," says Dr. Sotile. Financial fears also come into play, especially if the husband is the main or only wage earner.

Offer help to a friend in need and accept the help if the situation is your own. That's what friends are for. When you offer your help, be specific about what you can do. A "Let me know if I can do something to help" will only elicit a "Thank you," but the offer of a specific service is more likely to get you a taker. It will also show that you're sincere.

Tip 88: **Find a Furry Friend**

Harry Truman once said, "If you want a friend in Washington, get a dog." When the late president made the remark way back when, he had no idea that he was dispensing smart heart-health advice, too.

It has been a few decades since medical science showed that pets can peak the happiness quotient—and therefore, the healing process—in sick people. Research has found, for example, that merely petting a dog can bring down high blood pressure. Many hospitals and nursing homes now have pet visiting hours because of the benefits it bestows on patients.

Researchers demonstrated the medical meaning of puppy love by using 48 male and female stockbrokers with high blood pressure as guinea pigs. The researchers intentionally reproduced two situations that mimicked the type of stress the brokers experience in a typical day: In the first test, they were ordered to rapidly count backward, and in the second they had to spontaneously talk their way out of a make-believe shoplifting charge. Collectively their already-high blood pressures shot up to 184/129. (Blood pressure above 140/90 is considered high.) All the brokers were given blood-pressure medication, and half agreed to get a cat or a dog.

Broken Heart Club

"Good grief! You nearly gave me a heart attack!"

There is a lot of truth in this old, worn out expression. Puzzled doctors at Johns Hopkins Medical Center in Baltimore figured this out by investigating a small number of mysterious heart attacks that were recorded at the hospital. Over the course of several months, 18 women (and a few men) were brought to the emergency room with common signs of a heart attack and admitted for treatment. Only thing was, they all recovered rather quickly and, on testing, they showed no signs of ever having had a heart attack. Their condition only mimicked a heart attack—but they were not play acting.

It turns out the women had been so stunned by shocking news that their bodies secreted stress hormones in quantities so large that they temporarily turned toxic. The toxic reaction—chest pain, sweating, and shortness of breath—was just like a heart attack. The shock that threw them in such a heightened state of anxiety included news of a death, a surprise party, an armed robbery, and a court appearance.

The doctors coined the bizarre condition Broken Heart Syndrome.

Six months later, they were called back to go through two other tests that simulated the stress in a broker's life, but this time, the pet owners had their Lassies and Tabbies by their sides. Sure enough, blood pressure zoomed, but the pet owners' pressure went up only half as much as their petless colleagues.

No surprise to the researchers. They weren't even surprised that most of the brokers decided to get a pet! It probably wouldn't have surprised Harry Truman either.

10 Be **Good** to Yourself

A few years ago, a major household products company con-
ducted a survey in which they asked women to rate their
responsibilities by order of importance in their lives. Here is how
it tallied out:

1 Kids

2 Home

3 Job/career

4 Family pet(s)

5 Spouse

6 Yourself

When Sharonne N. Hayes, M.D., shows this slide at
WomenHeart's annual leadership symposium, it elicits a few
chuckles and some serious nods. The pet before spouse, obvi
ously, gets the laughs, but the silent assenting nod is the sobering acknowledgement of where they see themselves—last in

their own order of importance. It's sobering because they recognize that it is one of the reasons they are together—a group of women in their forties, fifties, and sixties learning how to resume life after having a heart attack. They also have something else in common: They can't imagine putting themselves first. But it is one of the things they know they must learn.

"Women are too guilt-ridden to put themselves first, and they've gotten the message that they can't come in last. We tell them they have to move up to where they at least tie for first," says Nancy Loving, Executive Director of WomenHeart: The National Coalition for Women with Heart Disease.

Loving speaks from personal experience. She had a heart attack at age 48 and found herself angry over her ignorance that such a thing could happen. "Like a lot of women who have had a heart attack, I was caught blindsided and ended up alone at my own pity party wanting my old life back. Well, I found out you can't have your old life back, but you can have a new, *better* life," she says. That entails more than eating healthy and exercising regularly. It also means putting your heart health at the top of your list of personal responsibilities.

Even the women among us who understand the importance of healthy food and exercise are surprised to find out that tending to kids, spouse, parents, job, house, and any number of other responsibilities except ourselves is a blueprint for a heart attack.

This isn't a message just for women who have had a heart attack. It is also for women who want to avoid one. The number-one take-home message from every expert who contributed to this book was the same: Women need to take better care of themselves.

DOING A 180

> "I've always catered to everyone's feelings but my own. I guess this is a common characteristic among women and all the more reason we need a place to focus on our emotional needs." —Tapati, diagnosed with heart disease at age 42

Sound like you? As selfless and altruistic as it is and however much appreciated it is by your loved ones, it also can be your own undoing. This is especially true if you are one of the eight million women in the United States who knows she has heart disease. So, file away the guilt and step into a new style of living.

Admit it. No one deserves it more than you.

Something Has to Change

You'd think that a woman who goes through a life-threatening illness such as a heart attack would see the future as a second chance to get more out of life. Rather, they mostly feel anxiety over disrupting life at home.

"They return too quickly to their domestic responsibilities and don't take care of themselves properly," says Nancy Loving of WomenHeart. "They feel the pressure from their families wanting their lives to return to normal, too." In WomenHeart's first-ever national survey on women with heart disease conducted in 2003, 27 percent said their relationships with their families had deteriorated because they could not adequately perform their duties at home.

Tip 89: Take Time for Yourself

Take 30 minutes of family or home time for yourself every day. Your lunch break from work does not apply. "This should be your quiet time," says Loving. "Read a book, listen to music, do nothing. Do whatever it is you want to do. Let your family know that this is your time, and it is not negotiable."

The idea, she says, is to relax. "Women who end up with heart attacks don't take time to relax. They are too busy being all things to all people. Whether you want to prevent another heart attack or the first one, this has to change."

Make your own space. If you have a room in your home that is not used often, make it your room. Decorate it just for you and fill it with the things you love. Let others know that if they use your room when you are not around, you expect them to leave it the way they found it.

Tip 90: Buy Yourself Time

Doing for yourself requires that you have the time to do it. The obvious approach, of course, is delegating some of your responsibilities to others in the household. That's a start, but what about the chores you just hate?

Delegate smartly. You don't want to delegate something to someone who hates it just as much as you, but you might be able to pay someone to do the job. Many women, for example, love gardening and find cultivating flowers nurturing and therapeutic. Some women love gardens but hate the digging and the dirt. If a lawn service is too hard on your budget, consider other ways to get someone else to do the work. Many communities have colleges or technical schools where students study horticulture or similar subjects. Perhaps one would be interested in taking on your yard as a project. The idea is to be creative in coming up with ways to take some of the burden off of yourself.

Take a clean break. The obvious way to help buy yourself time is to hire someone to help with the housework. Consider having someone in to clean. Even monthly is better than never. Perhaps you could pay someone to do the laundry or the ironing. Your health is certainly worth the money. Or, put another way, paying for help is better than spending the money on medication or doctor bills.

Tip 91: Pamper Yourself with Little Pleasures

"Soothe yourself every day in some small way by doing something that makes you feel good," says Loving. This could be having a manicure or a massage, buying yourself a pair of shoes you don't really need, or getting your hair done just for the heck of it.

After her heart attack, Loving had to learn to slow down and get to know herself better. She found that doing something that gave her pleasure also had the added benefit of making her feel more relaxed. Some things have become a ritual. "Every Saturday morning, I go out and buy three bouquets of flowers for the house," she says. A bit indulgent? Maybe. But that's the whole idea!

Tip 92: Be Spontaneous

Does it seem like everybody else is having fun and you're not? Then join the fun once in a while and don't allow anyone to let you feel guilty about it. If you want to meet a girlfriend for a glass of wine after work, or feel like seeing a movie all by yourself, call home and tell the family to have dinner without you. For a change, you can be the one to call and say that you won't be making it home for dinner. You might even want to add, "and don't wait up."

Every once in a while, you need to say to yourself, "What the

Been There, Done That

Age 65, so we're told, is the new 45. So keep this in mind next time you assume grandmother is eager for child-care duties.

When Harvard Medical School researchers analyzed more than 30 years of data from the Nurses' Health Study they accidentally came upon an interesting discovery: Women who spent as few as 9 hours a week caring for grandchildren increased their risk of heart disease by 55 percent.

The finding was distilled from the questionnaires filled out by 54,000 registered nurses who were free of heart disease, stroke, or cancer. During the following 4 years, 321 of them had heart attacks. After statistically adjusting for heart disease factors such as high cholesterol and blood pressure, they found that these women had one thing most in common: caring for their grandchildren at least 9 hours a week.

"It is possible that women, especially grandmothers with high levels of child-care demands, have less opportunity to engage in their own self-care and in preventive health behaviors," reported the researchers. Other studies have shown that care-giving grandmothers also are more likely to be depressed than other grandmothers. Researchers speculate that they simply may not have enough time to enjoy their own lives.

heck, why not!" and give yourself permission, says Loving. It's self-empowering and it will give your mood and ego a lift.

Tip 93: **Have a Night Out with the Girls**

As mentioned in Chapter 9, studies show that having a network of friends is practically a health requirement for women. Join a book club, a bridge game, a gourmet group, or just have a monthly dinner date with a good friend. Form a girls' group with friends who have common interests. Take a class or get involved in a hobby you enjoy. These are great ways to meet new women who share a common interest.

Make it a weekend. Men have been doing it for years in the name of sports—golfing, hunting, fishing, and going to football games. Find a small place to rent around some event you and your girlfriends will enjoy, perhaps an antique show or a play. Or just spend a weekend dedicated to healthy indulgence—cooking great food, drinking a little wine, spending a few hours at a day spa.

Tip 94: **Make a Little Dream Come True**

Every woman has an "I wish I would have..." or an "I've always wanted to..." list of dreams filed away in her mind. Shake those thoughts loose and get them down on paper. Some have gone unfulfilled because of money, but it's likely there are plenty of things you put off because you didn't have the time. Pick something that is attainable and will improve your life in some way. Then take action to make your dream come true.

> *"I am still not great about taking care of myself. But I did learn that it's okay to slip on the satin bed jacket and ask for help. In fact, you have to."* — Susan, age 41

Doing things that are good for you should not be once-in-awhile pleasures; they should happen every day. Think about your daily routine. Where do everyday tasks like getting up and going to bed rank on your pleasure barometer? If they are not near the top, you need to turn it up a few notches. Starting and ending your day in style should be part of your daily relaxation ritual.

Tip 95: Treat Yourself to the Perfect Bath

Aromatherapy expert and holistic nurse Valerie Gennari Cooksley, R.N., believes that the greatest way to relax and unwind at the end of the day is with a long meditative, aromatic soak. "In today's stressful and fast-paced world, we rarely allow ourselves enough time for a quick shower in the morning, let alone an indulgent, relaxing bath," she says. "Ironically, the women who say they haven't the time for such a luxury are the ones who really need it the most."

A bath in and of itself will have a relaxing effect, but adding essential oils to the bath and placing some relaxing scents in the room will make you feel like you've had the entire day off, she says.

To get the most pleasure out of your bath, there are two things you have to get right: the water temperature and the essential oils. Make sure the bath water is warm, not hot. The ideal temperature should be between 92° and 100°F. Bath water that makes you perspire is too hot. It also is not good if you have high blood pressure because it will make your heart rate go up for a few minutes. So be cautious. (Until you learn how the desired water temperature should feel to your touch, you can check the temperature using a thermometer.)

Before you get in the bath, add a few drops of an essential oil that is known to bring calm and relaxation. These include chamomile, lemon verbena, lemon balm, lavender, and rose. Not only do they smell wonderful, says Cooksley, but they will make your skin feel smooth.

Add some spa accents. Turn down the lights, light a few candles. Throw some rose petals into the water to add to the indulgence. If

Stay Snug and Warm in Winter

Hate the bitter cold? If you have heart disease, you have a great excuse to stay cozy and warm indoors. Winter is the top season for heart attacks, followed by fall, spring, then summer. Winter heart attacks also tend to be more serious and result in more damage to the heart than in any other season.

Women with high blood pressure are more vulnerable to heart attacks when the temperature drops below 39.3°F and also when the temperature drops more than 9 degrees in a single day, regardless of how cold it is. The reason is because hearts have to work harder in winter. In the cold, blood flow to the periphery of the body decreases to conserve body heat. Narrowed vessels put more strain on the heart. Also cholesterol levels are higher in winter, especially in women.

that seems too over the top, you can peel the zest from fresh oranges, grapefruit, or lemons and let it float in the bath water. All will add a refreshing fragrance.

Next, wrap your hair in a towel, get in the tub, submerge yourself to your neck, lean back, and close your eyes. This will get you in a meditative state. "Focus your attention on your thoughts, then gradually create a space between your thoughts and the outside world," suggests Cooksley.

Concentrate on your breathing by inhaling deeply and slowly. Exhale through your nose, pushing out all the day's stress and negative energy.

Tip 96: Make Sleep a Priority

Sleep is like a dimmer switch for the heart. While you sleep, heart rate slows and blood pressure relaxes to the lowest point of the day. When you spend a night tossing and turning, however, your heart doesn't get a time-out, so it will beat faster for a longer period of time during the course of a day. Blood pressure that should be relaxing must work harder, meaning the day's average pressure will be higher than it would be if you got a restful night's sleep.

Women, unfortunately, do not give sleep the respect it deserves. First, most of us do not get enough sleep. Working women between the ages of 30 and 60 get an average of only 6 hours and 41 minutes of sleep a night during the work week, according to statistics. Doctors say most women need 8 hours a night. On top of that, a lot of us are not getting quality sleep. Statistics show that 63 percent of women, compared to 52 percent of men, complain of insomnia at least a few times a week.

Bad sleep takes a toll. One study that followed 71,617 women between the ages of 45 and 65 for 10 years found that those who routinely slept less than 8 hours a night had an increased risk for heart attack and heart-related death. Among them, those who got 5 or fewer hours a night ended up with higher blood pressure, cholesterol, and blood sugar that increased their risk of getting a heart attack by 45 percent.

One thing that interferes with sleep is our biology. The hormonal shifts of menstruation, pregnancy, and menopause can disturb the deep stage of sleep known as REM (rapid eye movement). For example, sleep experts say women report disturbed sleep 2 to 3 days before the start of their periods. More than half of women going through menopause report interrupted sleep due to hot flashes. This is the

A Really Bad Day Remedy
When stress reaches epidemic proportions, aromatherapist and holistic nurse Valerie Gennari Cooksley, R.N., recommends taking a body-temperature bath (about 98°F) in complete darkness. "It's a great antidote for stress-caused sensory overload," she says.

"By making the bath water the same temperature as your body, you create a sense of sensory deprivation as the nerve endings in your skin become desensitized," she explains. You'll sense neither hot nor cold. "Just be ready for a profound experience!" she says.

time in her life when a woman can develop snoring and sleep apnea, a disruption in breathing that breaks the sleep cycle. Experts report that this develops in one out of every four women over the age of 65.

Sleep like a baby. "Sleep should not be considered a luxury but an important component of a healthy lifestyle," reported the researchers in the sleep study.

To get in the habit of a good night's sleep, experts say you should go to bed at the same time each night and get up 8 hours later. To help you sleep, they recommend that you:

- ❤ Avoid food, caffeine, and alcohol within a few hours of bedtime.

- ❤ Exercise early in the day, if possible, and never within 3 to 4 hours of bedtime. One study found that post-menopausal women who exercise in the morning experience less difficulty falling asleep.

- ❤ Keep distractions like television, work, and desks filled with bills out of the bedroom.

How Much Is Too Much?

Too much sleep can be just as bad for your heart as too little. At least that is what the results of one study indicates. The study, which followed 71,617 women for 10 years, found that women who regularly slept 9 or more hours a night had a 38 percent greater risk of getting a heart attack than women who got 7 to 8 hours.

♥ Keep the temperature in your bedroom slightly cooler than you do in the rest of the house.

♥ Have a comfortable mattress and a pillow that supports your head so it remains aligned with your spine when lying on your side.

♥ Do not nap during the day.

Tip 97: Make like a Tree and Sleep

You don't have to have the flexibility of a gymnast to benefit from the relaxing art of yoga. Yoga is a centuries-old discipline of relaxation poses designed to stimulate internal organs and nerves to either invigorate or induce a meditative state. "Yoga releases the day's tension and can draw you from a hectic stressed-induced life into a quiet, peaceful interlude," says Cooksley. Yoga has the added benefit of stretching and strengthening muscles and achieving balance.

Yoga requires that you fully concentrate on the pose, which in turn relaxes the mind and encourages rhythmic breathing. Cooksley recommends doing the tree pose before climbing into bed. Concentrating on the pose as you are doing it, says Cooksley, will relax your mind and encourage slow and even breathing.

The tree pose is a little difficult at first, but you should get the hang of it quickly. Stand by the side of the bed to help you with your balance. You'll feel a nice stretch as you do this:

♥ Stand with your feet shoulder-width apart. Relax your head and look straight ahead. Relax your knees and shift your weight to your right leg.

♥ Stretch your arms out from your body for balance and turn your left knee and foot out to the side. Bring your heel towards your right ankle.

♥ Slide your left foot up the inside of your right calf, then to your inner thigh where it will rest. Move your left knee backward and your left hip forward.

♥ When you feel the balance, bring your arms toward your chest and put your palms together in a prayer position. Inhale deeply and slowly exhale.

The Coffee Catch

Is coffee bad for the heart, or isn't it? The answer appears to be neither, as long as you keep your quota to a cup or two a day, especially if you have heart disease.

One study of 3,000 residents in Greece, however, found that those who drink moderate to high amounts of coffee had signs of ongoing low levels of inflammation, a marker for the development of heart disease. Those who did not drink coffee did not.

The bottom line? "We do not specifically advise for or against the consumption of coffee or other caffeinated drinks," says the American Heart Association.

- ♥ Keeping your palms together, raise your arms straight up and overhead. Breathe deeply six times.

- ♥ Bring your arms and leg back to position by reversing the order of movement. Repeat on other side.

Tip 98: Take Time for Tea

Sit, relax, sip tea, and enjoy a moment of bliss.

This is what Miriam Novalle wants from everyone who walks into The T Salon, the comfy emporium she operates in the Chelsea section of New York City. "Taking tea provides a precious timeout from a busy schedule. Allow tea and faith to elevate your spirit," she writes on her menu. And, she could add, strengthen your heart.

Coffeehouses and coffee drinking are the far more American way to relax, but they have nothing to offer your health or your heart. No so for tea. Tea, in fact, shares the same rare heart healthy properties that are found in red wine.

The magic of tea is found in polyphenols. These phytonutrients are so abundant that they make up 30 percent of tea's dry weight. Green tea gets most of the good press, but in truth, any tea is good for your heart. Green is simply the least processed of the three, but black and oolong are just as healthy.

Going exotic goes way beyond Earl Grey and Darjeeling. Tea comes in such an infinite number of varieties and flavors, you could experiment with something different almost every day. The T Salon, for example, offers more than 150 selections.

When you take a break, think tea. Unlike coffee, you'll get a bit of health with every sip.

Tip 99: Shine a Winning Smile

A great grin is a sign that you're happy—that's important!—but it is also a sign of good dental health. If you don't have teeth and gums you can smile about, you should visit your dentist. Maintaining good dental health is important to your heart, because research has found an association between gum disease and heart disease.

The focus of concern is periodontal disease, a totally avoidable and painful bacterial infection of the gums that, left untreated, can lead to tooth loss. In one study, for example, 657 people who developed periodontal disease but had no history of having a heart attack or a stroke were found to have thickening of the carotid artery—the main artery that transports blood to the head and brain—equal to the levels of bacteria in their bodies.

Doctors believe that the bacteria can travel through the bloodstream to the arteries and trigger a cycle of inflammation that can lead to heart disease. They also believe it can make you more prone to high blood pressure and blood clots. And research indicates that women with periodontal disease are almost twice as likely to have a fatal heart attack as women with healthy gums.

The link to heart disease is strong enough that it is considered an identifiable risk by the American Academy of Periodontology.

Keep your dentist in the know. The Academy says that if you have heart disease, you should let your dentist know. Dental procedures, even routine visits, have the tendency to raise blood pressure and heart rates.

It's best to schedule your appointment for first thing in the morning when blood pressure is at its lowest and before any of the stresses of life have a chance to work you up. One study at the

University of Bologna in Italy found that heart disease patients with blood pressure that is adversely affected by stress could be at risk for heart failure in the dentist's chair.

Floss and brush. The best way to protect your teeth is to floss and brush your teeth as if your life depended on it. Hint: brushing action and the right toothbrush are more important than the kind of toothpaste you use, say dentists. Your toothbrush should be soft so that it can get in and around every tooth. Always floss first. Your dental ritual should take 3 to 5 minutes twice a day.

Tip 100: **Breathe a Lot of Fresh Air**

It's long been known that constant exposure to air pollution can lead to lung damage, but there is now evidence that it can be harmful to your heart. Though the risk is relatively small compared with established risk factors, it is concern enough to get the attention of the American Heart Association. The source of concern is particulate matter, the type of grime caused by automobile emissions, road dust, power generation, industrial smelting, metal processing, construction and demolition sites, wood-burning fireplaces, and pollen and molds, just to name a few. Research shows that when we inhale ultrafine particles, they enter the bloodstream and can thicken the blood and boost inflammation.

According to at least one study, older women appear to be most vulnerable to the ill-effects of air pollution. The long-term study, conducted on 798 men and women in the smoggy Los Angeles area, found that those exposed to the most air pollution over the years had the most buildup of plaque in their carotid artery. Those with the least exposure had the least thickening of the artery. In women over age 60, the arterial thickening was four times the average of all 800. Second to women, those most vulnerable to damage from air pollution were nonsmokers and people who take drugs to lower cholesterol.

Here are some measures you can take to minimize your exposure to air pollution:

Avoid going outdoors when the air is bad. The EPA provides daily information about ozone and particulate matter levels for more than 150 cities. Daily newspapers in these areas usually post a pollution report. You can find out about the air quality in your area by logging onto www.epa.gov/airnow.

Stay out of smoke-filled rooms. Secondhand smoke is believed to contribute to 35,000 deaths in the United States each year. Studies have shown that secondhand smoke can increase heart disease risk in nonsmokers by an estimated 25 percent, but a recent study in the United Kingdom indicates the number may be even higher. This study found that nonsmokers with the highest blood levels of cotinine, a by-product of nicotine in cigarette smoke, had a 50 percent higher risk of heart disease than those with the lowest levels of cotinine in their blood.

"We have known for some time that passive smoking was strongly associated with increased risk of coronary heart disease, but this study strengthens the evidence," reported Tom Bowker, M.D., a physician with the British Heart Foundation.

Work and play in a smoke-free environment. The smoke from even one smoker is enough to pollute a room and is the single largest contributor to indoor air pollution. Most work environments are smoke-free and many states and even some countries (like the Republic of Ireland) have banned smoking in public places. You have the freedom of choice, so choose to surround yourself with the cleanest air possible.

Make your home a smoke-free zone. Most guests who smoke understand this rule and do not take it as an affront. A smoking member of your family may feel differently, but stand your ground. By forcing smokers outdoors, you are helping them cut back.

Tip 101: **Speak Up for Your Health**

Are you satisfied with your health care? Is your doctor willing to listen to your concerns and take them seriously? If your answer on both counts is "No," you have a lot of company.

When WomenHeart did its national health-care survey, more than half of the women with heart disease said they were dissatisfied with some aspect of their health care. Specifically, 58 percent said they did not like their physicians' attitudes and communication styles. They used words like insensitive, rude, abrupt, and ignorant about heart disease in women. It's an attitude they are trying to help change.

Empower yourself. Women need to be diligent about their heart health, be aware of the symptoms of heart disease, report anything unusual to their doctors, and be assertive about getting diagnostic tests if their concerns are brushed off. "Only 35 percent of the women in our survey recognized their symptoms as heart-related, and 45 percent felt their heart disease came out of the blue," says WomenHeart's Nancy Loving. "They end up as patients who feel confused, ignored, and don't know what questions to ask."

The National Coalition of Women with Heart Disease wants to see this change. Each year, more women are becoming aware that heart disease is the number-one killer of women worldwide. A recent poll found the number has doubled since 2000.

We are a lot slower, however, in accepting it as a personal threat. The same poll found that women are still more concerned about breast cancer. Perhaps this is due, at least in part, to the notion that protecting ourselves against heart disease means sacrificing a part of our individual lifestyles.

To the contrary, protecting your heart can enhance your lifestyle. Think about it and picture yourself: sipping a glass of wine... nibbling a little chocolate... eating berries, avocados and other wonderfully fresh and tasty fruits... enjoying asparagus, sweet potatoes and other garden treats... experimenting with new and healthy foods... feeling refreshed and invigorated from a healthy walk or workout... leaving stress behind and enjoying the company of people who make you happy... and last, but certainly not least, making sure to make a little time for yourself every day.

References

Chapter 1

American Heart Association. 2005. *Heart Disease and Stroke Statistics—2005 Update.*

Emslie, C. 2005. Women, men and coronary heart disease: a review of the qualitative literature. *Journal of Advanced Nursing.* Aug.; 51(4):382-95.

Gerstenblith, G., Margolis, S. 2004. *The Johns Hopkins White Papers, Coronary Heart Disease—2004.*

Goldberb, Neica, M.D. 2002. *Women Are Not Small Men.* Ballantine Books.

Grace, S.L. et al. 2003. Presentation, delay, and contraindication to thrombolytic treatment in females and males with myocardial infarction. *Women's Health Issues.* Nov.-Dec.; 13(6):214-21

Jacobs, A.K., Eckel, R.H. 2005. Evaluating and managing cardiovascular disease in women: understanding a woman's heart. *Circulation.* Feb. 1; 111(4):383-84.

Johnson, P.A., Manson, J.E. 2005. Cardiology patient page. How to make sure the beat goes on: protecting a woman's heart. Feb. 1; 111(4):e28-33.

Kromhout D., et al. 2002. Prevention of coronary heart disease by diet and lifestyle: evidence from prospective cross-cultural, cohort, and intervention studies. *Circulation.* Feb. 19; 105(7):893-98.

Lagato, Marianne J., M.D. 2003. *Eve's Rib: The Groundbreaking Guide to Women's Health.* Three Rivers Press.

Miers, J.H. et al. 2005. Role of noninvasive testing in the clinical evaluation of women with suspected coronary artery disease: consensus statement from the Cardiac Imaging Committee, Council on Clinical Cardiology, and the Cardiovascular Imaging and Intervention Committee, Council on Cardiovascular Radiology and Intervention, American Heart Association, *Circulation.* Feb. 8; 111(5):682-96.

Martin, R. et al. 2004. Gender disparities in common sense models of illness among myocardial infarction victims, *Health Psychology*, July; 23(4):345-53.

Mosca, L. et al. 2005. National study of physician awareness and adherence to cardiovascular disease prevention guidelines, *Circulation*, Feb. 1; 111(4):499-510.

Mosca, L., et al. 2004. Tracking women's awareness of heart disease: an American Heart Association national study. *Circulation.* Feb. 10; 109(5):573-79.

Mosca, L., et al. 2004. Evidence-based guidelines for cardiovascular disease prevention in women. *Circulation.* Feb. 10; 109(5):672-93.

Patel H. et al. 2004. Symptoms in acute coronary syndromes: does sex make a difference? *American Heart Journal.* July; 148(1):27-33.

Selvin, E., Erlinger, T.P. 2004. Prevalence of and risk factors for peripheral arterial disease in the United States: results from the National Health and Nutrition Examination Survey, 1999-2000, *Circulation*, Aug. 10; 110(6):738-43.

Spertus, J.A., et al. 2005. American College of Cardiology and American Heart Association methodology for the selection and creation of performance measures for quantifying the quality of cardiovascular care. *Journal of the American College of Cardiology.* April 5; 45(7):1147-56.

Chapter 2

Anthonisen, N.R., et al. 2005. The effects of a smoking cessation intervention on 14.5-year mortality: a randomized clinical trial. *Annals of Internal Medicine.* Feb. 15; 142(4):112.

Ambrose J.A., Barua, R.S. 2004. The pathophysiology of cigarette smoking and cardiovascular disease: an update. *Journal of the American College of Cardiology* May 19; 43(10):1731-37.

American Heart Association. 2005. *Heart Disease and Stroke Statistics— 2005 Update.*

American Lung Association. 2004. *Women and Smoking Fact Sheet.*

Canzanello, V.J., et al. 2005. Improved blood pressure control with a physician-nurse team and home blood pressure measurement. *Mayo Clinic Proceedings.* Jan.; 80(1):19.

Chen W., et al. 2005. Metabolic syndrome variables at low levels in childhood are beneficially associated with adulthood cardiovascular risk: the Bogalusa Heart Study. *Diabetes Care.* Jan.; 28(1):126-31.

Dagenais, G.R., et al. 2005. Prognostic impact of body weight and abdominal obesity in women and men with cardiovascular disease. *American Heart Journal.* Jan.; 149(1):54-60.

Eisenmann, J.C., et al. 2005. Relationship between adolescent fitness and fatness and cardiovascular disease risk factors in adulthood: the Aerobics Center Longitudinal Study. *American Heart Journal.* Jan.; 149(1):46-53.

Ezzati, M., et al. 2005. Role of smoking in global and regional cardiovascular mortality. *Circulation.* July 26; 112(4):489-97.

Fields, L.E., et al. 2004. The burden of adult hypertension in the
United States 1999 to 2000: a rising tide. *Hypertension.* Oct.;
44(4):389.

Fischer, M., et al. 2005. Distinct heritable patterns of angiographic
coronary artery disease in families with myocardial infarction.
Circulation. Feb. 22; 111(7):855-62.

Gerstenblith, G., Margolis, S. 2004. *The Johns Hopkins White Papers,
Coronary Heart Disease—2004.*

Gunderson, E.P., et al. 2004. Long-term plasma lipid changes associated with a first birth: the Coronary Artery Risk Development in
Young Adults study. *American Journal of Epidemiology,* June 1;
159(11):1028-39.

Inoue, T., et al. 2005. Local release of C-reactive protein from vulnerable plaque or coronary arterial wall injured by stenting. *Journal
of the American College of Cardiology.* July 19; 46(2):239-45.

Johnsen, S.H., et al. 2005. Elevated high-density lipoprotein cholesterol levels are protective against plaque progression: a follow-up
study of 1952 persons with carotid atherosclerosis the Tromso
study. *Circulation.* July 26; 112(4):498-504.

Levantesi, G., et al. 2005. Metabolic syndrome and risk of cardiovascular events after myocardial infarction. *Journal of the American
College of Cardiology.* July 19; 46(2):277-83.

Mahonen, M.S., et al. 2004. Current smoking and the risk of nonfatal myocardial infarction in the WHO MONICA Project popula-
tions. *Tobacco Control,* Sept.; 13(3):244-50.

2001. *Mayo Clinic Women's Healthsource.* Dec.; 5(12):1-2.

Miranda, P.J., et al. 2005. Metabolic syndrome: definition, pathophysiology, and mechanisms. *American Heart Journal.* Jan.;
149(1):33-45.

Montonen, J., et al. 2005. Dietary patterns and the incidence of type 2 diabetes. *American Journal of Epidemiology*. Feb. 1; 161(3):219-27.

Mosca, L., et al. 2005. Opportunity for intervention to achieve American Heart Association guidelines for optimal lipid levels in high-risk women in a managed care setting. *Circulation*, Feb. 1; 111(4):488-93.

Pickering, T.G., et al. 2005. Recommendations for blood pressure measurement in humans and experimental animals: Part 1: blood pressure measurement in humans: a statement for professionals from the Subcommittee of Professional and Public Education of the American Heart Association Council on High Blood Pressure Research. *Hypertension*. May; 45(5):15.

Pokorny, S.B., et al. 2004. Current smoking among young adolescents: assessing school based contextual norms. *Tobacco Control*. Sept.; 13(3):301-7.

Rossi, E., et al. 2002. Risk of myocardial infarction and angina in patients with severe peripheral vascular disease: predictive role of C-reactive protein. *Circulation*. Feb. 19; 105(7):800-3.

Rutter, M.K. et al.2004. C-reactive protein, the metabolic syndrome, and prediction of cardiovascular events in the Framingham Offspring Study, *Circulation*. July 27; 110(4):380-85.

Samet, J.M. 2005. Smoking kills: experimental proof from the Lung Health Study. *Annals of Internal Medicine*. Feb. 15; 142(4):299-301.

Saudek, C.D., Margolis, S. 2004. *The Johns Hopkins White Papers*, *Diabetes—2004*.

Twardella, D., et al. 2004. Short-term benefit of smoking cessation in patients with coronary heart disease: estimates based on self-reported smoking data and serum cotinine measurements. *European Heart Journal*. Dec.; 25(23):2101-8.

Vitarius, J.A. The metabolic syndrome and cardiovascular disease. *Mount Sinai Journal of Medicine*. July; 72(4):257-62.

Chapter 3

Dell'Agli M., et al. 2004. Vascular effects of wine polyphenols, *Cardiovascular Research*. Sept. 1; 63(4): 593-602.

Djousse, L., et al. 2004. Alcohol consumption and metabolic syndrome: does the type of beverage matter? *Obesity Research*. Sept.; 12(9):13075-85.

Ellison, R.C., et al. 2004. Lifestyle determinants of high-density lipoprotein cholesterol: the National Heart, Lung, and Blood Institute Family Heart Study. *American Heart Journal*. March; 147(3):529-35.

Ellison, R.C. 2002. Balancing the risks and benefits of moderate drinking. *Annals of the New York Academy of Science*. May; 957:1-6.

Engler, M.B., et al. 2004. Flavonoid-rich dark chocolate improves endothelial function and increases plasma epicatechin concentrations in healthy adults. *Journal of the American College of Nutrition*. June; 23(3):197-204.

Fraga, C. 2005. Cocoa, diabetes, and hypertension: should we eat more chocolate? *American Journal of Clinical Nutrition*. March; 81(3):541-42.

Fuhrman, B. et al. 2001. White wine with red wine-like properties: increased extraction of grape skin polyphenols improves the antioxidant capacity of the derived white wine. *Journal of Agriculture and Food Chemistry*. July; 49(7):3164-8.

Glaser, J.H. 2000. Why mortality from heart disease is low in France. Wine consumption clearly correlates with residual differences in mortality. *British Medical Journal*. Jan. 22; 320(7229):250.

Grassi, D., et al. 2005. Cocoa reduces blood pressure and insulin resistance and improves endothelium-dependent vasodilation in hypertensives. *Hypertension*. Aug.; 46(2):398-405.

Grassi, D., et al. 2005. Short-term administration of dark chocolate is followed by a significant increase in insulin sensitivity and a decrease in blood pressure in healthy persons. *American Journal of Clinical Nutrition*. March; 81(3):611-14.

Greenfield, J.R., et al. 2005. Beneficial postprandial effect of a small amount of alcohol on diabetes and cardiovascular risk factors: modification by insulin resistance. *Journal of Clinical Endocrinology and Metabolism*. Feb.; 90(2):661-72.

Gronbaek, M., Sorensen, T.L. 1996. Alcohol consumption and risk of coronary heart disease. Studies suggest that wine has additional effect to that of ethanol. *British Medical Journal*. March 23; 312(7033):731-6.

Imhof, A., et al. 2004. Overall alcohol intake, beer, wine, and systemic markers of inflammation in western Europe; results from three MONICA samples (Augsburg, Glasgow, Lille). *European Heart Journal*. Dec.; 25(23):2075-76.

Karatzi, K., et al. 2004 Constituents of red wine other than alcohol improve endothelial function in patients with coronary artery disease. *Coronary Artery Disease*. Dec.15; (8):485-90.

Klatsky. A.L., et al. 2005. Alcohol drinking and risk of hospitalization for heart failure with and without coronary artery disease, *American Journal of Cardiology*. Aug. 1; 96(3):346-51.

Kondo, K., et al. 1996. Inhibition of LDL oxidation by cocoa, *Lancet*. Nov 30; 348(9040).

Koppes. L., et al. 2005. Moderate alcohol consumption lowers the risk of type 2 diabetes: a meta-analysis of prospective observational studies. *Diabetes Care*. March; 28(3):719-25.

Mursu, J., et al. 2004. Dark chocolate consumption increases HDL cholesterol concentration and chocolate fatty acids may inhibit lipid peroxidation in healthy humans. *Free Radical Biology and Medicine*. Nov. 1; 37(9):1351-9.

Perez-Magarino, S., Gonzalez-San Jose., M.L. 2004. Evolution of flavanols, anthocyanins, and their derivatives during the aging of red
wines elaborated from grapes harvested at different stages of
ripening. *Journal of Agriculture and Food Chemistry*. March 10;
52(5):1181-89.

Rimm, E.B., et al. 1996. Review of moderate alcohol consumption
and reduced risk of coronary heart disease: is the effect due to
beer, wine, or spirits. *British Medical Journal*. March 23;
312(7033):731-6.

Tjonneland, A., et al. 1999. Wine intake and diet in a random sample of 48763 Danish men and women. *American Journal of Clinical
Nutrition*. Jan.; 69(1):2-3.

Vlachopoulos, C., et al. 2005. Effect of dark chocolate on arterial
function in healthy individuals. *American Journal of Hypertension*.
June; 18(6):785-91.

Wan, Y., et al. 2001. Effects of cocoa powder and dark chocolate on
LDL oxidative susceptibility and prostaglandin concentrations in
humans. *American Journal of Clinical Nutrition*. Nov.; 74(5):596-602.

Chapter 4

Almario, R.U., et al. 2001. Effects of walnut consumption on plasma
fatty acids and lipoproteins in combined hyperlipidemia. *American
Journal of Clinical Nutrition*. July; 74(1):72-9.

Berkow, S.E., Barnard, N.D. 2005. Blood pressure regulation and vegetarian diets. *Nutrition Reviews*. Jan.; 63(1):1-8.

Bray, G.A., et al. 2004. A further subgroup analysis of the effects of
the DASH diet and three dietary sodium levels on blood pressure:
results of the DASH-Sodium Trial. *The American Journal of Cardiology*.
July 15; 94(2):222-7.

Cereda, E., et al. 2005. Modified Mediterranean diet and survival:

evidence for diet linked longevity is substantial. *British Medical Journal.* April 30; 330(7498):991.

Cheysohoou, C., et al. 2004. Adherence to the Mediterranean diet attenuates inflammation and coagulation process in healthy adults: The ATTICA Study. *Journal of the American College of Cardiology.* July 7; 44(1):152-8.

Cordain L., et al. 2005. Origins and evolution of the Western diet: health implications for the 21st century. *The American Journal of Clinical Nutrition.* Feb.; 81(2):341-54.

Coulston, A.M. 1999. The role of dietary fats in plant-based diets. *The American Journal of Clinical Nutrition.* Sept.; 70(3):512S-515S.

Fennessy, F.M., et al. 2003. Taurine and vitamin C modify monocyte and endothelial dysfunction in young smokers. *Circulation.* Jan. 28; 107(3):410-5.

Franco, O.H., et al. 2004. The Polymeal: a more natural, safer, and probably tastier (than the Polypill) strategy to reduce cardiovascular disease by more than 75 percent. *British Medical Journal.* Dec. 18; 329(7480):1447-50.

Fung T., et al. 2004. Prospective study of major dietary patterns and stroke risk in women. *Stroke.* Sept.; 35(9):2014-9.

Ganji, V., Kafai, M.R. 2004. Frequent consumption of milk, yogurt, cold breakfast cereals, peppers, and cruciferous vegetables and intakes of dietary folate and riboflavin but not vitamins B_{12} and B_6 are inversely associated with serum total homocysteine concentrations in the U.S. population. *The American Journal of Clinical Nutrition.* Dec.; 80(6):1500-7.

Hu, F., et al. 2003. The Mediterranean diet and mortality—olive oil and beyond. *New England Journal of Medicine.* June 26; 348(26):2595-6.

Hu, F.B., et al. 2002. Fish and omega-3 fatty acid intake and risk of coronary heart disease in women. *Journal of the American Medical Association.* April 10; 287(14):1815-21.

Jambazian, P.R., et al. 2005. Almonds in the diet simultaneously improve plasma alpha-tocopherol concentrations and reduce plasma lipids. *Journal of the American Dietetic Association.* March; 105(3):449-54.

Jenkins, D.J., et al. 2005. Direct comparison of dietary portfolio vs. statin on C-reactive protein. *The American Journal of Clinical Nutrition.* Feb.; 81(2):380-7.

Jenkins, D.J., et al. 2003. Effects of a dietary portfolio of cholesterol-lowering foods vs. lovastatin on serum lipids and C-reactive protein. *Journal of the American Medical Association.* July 23; 290(4):502-10.

Juntunen. K.S., et al. High-fiber rye bread and insulin secretion and sensitivity in healthy postmenopausal women. *The American Journal of Clinical Nutrition.* Feb.; 77(2):385-91.

Katz, D.L., et al. 2005. Egg consumption and endothelial function: a randomized controlled crossover trial. *International Journal of Cardiology.* March 10; 99(1):65-70.

Kelemen, L.E., et al. 2005. Associations of dietary protein with disease and mortality in a prospective study of postmenopausal women. *American Journal of Epidemiology.* Feb.1; 161(3):239-49.

Kris-Etherton, P., et al. 1999. High-monounsaturated fatty acid diets lower both plasma cholesterol and triacylglycerol concentrations. *American Journal of Clinical Nutrition.* Dec.; 70(6):1009-15.

Kok, F.J., Kromhout, D. 2004. Atherosclerosis—epidemiological studies on the health effects of a Mediterranean diet. *European Journal of Nutrition.* March.

Larsen, L., et al. 1999. Are olive oil diets antithrombotic? Diets enriched with olive, rapeseed, or sunflower oil affect postprandial factor VII differently. *American Journal of Clinical Nutrition.* Dec.; 70(6):976-82.

Liu, S., et al. 1999. Whole-grain consumption and risk of coronary heart disease: results of the Nurses' Health Study. *The American Journal of Clinical Nutrition*. Sept.; 70(3):412-9.

Mayo Clinic Women's Healthsource. 2005. Eating fish. Getting the benefits, cutting the risks. Feb.; 9(2):7.

Mozaffarian, D., et al. 2004. Fish intake and risk of incident atrial fibrillation. *Circulation*. July 27; 110(4):368-73.

Thomsen, C., et al. 1999. Differential effects of saturated and monounsaturated fatty acids on postprandial lipemia and incretin responses in healthy subjects. *The American Journal of Clinical Nutrition*. June; 69(6):1135-43.

Panagiotakos, D.B., et al. 2005. Fish consumption and the risk of developing acute coronary syndromes: the CARDIO 2000 study. *International Journal of Cardiology*. July 20; 102(3):403-9.

Psaltopoulou, T., et al. 2004. Olive oil, the Mediterranean diet, and arterial blood pressure: the Greek European Prospective Investigation into Cancer and Nutrition (EPIC) study. *The American Journal of Clinical Nutrition*. Oct.; 80(4):1012-8.

Ros, E., et al. 2004. A walnut diet improves endothelial function in hypercholesterolemic subjects: a randomized crossover trial. *Circulation*. April 6; 109(13):1609-14.

Rosell, M.S., et al. 2004. Soy intake and blood cholesterol concentrations: a cross-sectional study of 1033 pre- and postmenopausal women in the Oxford arm of the European Prospective Investigation into Cancer and Nutrition. *The American Journal of Clinical Nutrition*. Nov.; 80(5):1391-6.

Trichopoulou A, Critselis, E. 2004. Mediterranean diet and longevity. *European Journal of Cancer Prevention*. Oct.; 13(5):453-56.

Yancy, W., et al. 2003. Diet and clinical coronary events. The truth is out there. *Circulation*. Jan.7; 107(1):10-6.

Chapter 5

American Heart Association. 2005. *Heart Disease and Stroke Statistics 2005 Update*. 48-51.

Bazzano, L.A., et al. 2002. Fruit and vegetable intake and risk of cardiovascular disease in U.S. adults: the first National Health and Nutrition Examination Survey Epidemiologic Follow-up Study. *The American Journal of Clinical Nutrition*. July; 76(1):1-2.

Clark, R. 2005. Homocysteine-lowering trials for prevention of heart disease and stroke. *Seminars in Vascular Medicine*. May; 5(2):215-22.

Craig, W.J. 1999. Health-promoting properties of common herbs. *The American Journal of Clinical Nutrition*. Sept.; 70(3):491S-99S.

Djousse, J. et al. 2004. Fruit and vegetable consumption and LDL cholesterol: the National Heart, Lung, and Blood Institute Family Heart Study. *The American Journal of Clinical Nutrition*, Feb.; 79(2):213-17.

Dutta-Roy, A.K., et al. 2002. Effects of tomato extract on human platelet aggregation in vitro. *Platelets*. June; 12(4):218-27.

George Mateljan Foundation. World's healthiest foods. *Whf.org*.

Hu, F.B. 2003. Plant-based foods and prevention of cardiovascular disease: an overview. *The American Journal of Clinical Nutrition*. Sept.; 78(3):544S-51S.

Kris-Etherton, P.M., et al. 2004. Antioxidant vitamin supplements and cardiovascular disease. *Circulation*. Aug. 3; 110(5):637-41.

Manach, C., et al. 2004. Polyphenols: food sources and bioavailability, *The American Journal of Clinical Nutrition*. May; 79(5)727-47.

Mazza, G. et al. 2002. Absorption of anthocyanins from blueberries and serum antioxidant status in human subjects. *Journal of Agriculture and Food Chemistry*. Dec. 18; 50(26):7731-37.

Miean, K.H., Mohamed, S. 2001.Flavonoid (myricetin, quercetin, kaempferol, luteolin, and apigenin) content of edible tropical plants. *Journal of Agricultural and Food Chemistry.* June; 49(6):3106-12.

Osganian, S.K., et al. 2003. Dietary carotenoids and risk of coronary artery disease in women. *The American Journal of Clinical Nutrition.* June; 77(6):1390-99.

Sesso, H.D., et al. 2004. Plasma lycopene, other carotenoids, and retinol and the risk of cardiovascular disease in women. *The American Journal of Clinical Nutrition.* Jan.; 79(1):47-53.

Chapter 6

American Heart Association. 2005. *Heart Disease and Stroke Statistics, Update 2005.* 37.

De Backer, G.G., De Bacquer, D. 2004. Be physically active: the best buy in promoting heart health. *European Heart Journal.* Dec.; 25(24):2183-4.

Blumenthal, J.A., et al. 2004. Exercise, depression, and mortality after myocardial infarction in the ENRICHD trial. *Medicine and Science in Sports and Exercise.* May; 36(5):746-55.

Carnethon, M.R., et al. Cardiorespiratory fitness in young adulthood and the development of cardiovascular disease risk factors. *Journal of the American Medical Association.* Dec. 17; 290(23):3092-100.

Dunn, A.L. et al. 2005. Exercise treatment for depression: efficacy and dose response. *American Journal of Preventive Medicine.* Jan.; 28(1):1-8.

Hillson, M.M., et al. 2005. Prospective study of physical activity and physical function in early old age. *American Journal of Preventive Medicine.* April; 28(3):245-50.

Lichtenstein, A.H. 1997. Trans fatty acids, plasma lipid levels, and risk of developing cardiovascular disease. A statement for health-care professionals from the American Heart Association. *Circulation.* June 3; 95(11):2588-90.

Mora, S. et al. 2003. Ability of exercise testing to predict cardiovascular and all-cause death in asymptomatic women: a 20-year follow-up of the lipid research clinics prevalence study. *Journal of the American Medical Association.* Sept. 24; 290(12):1600-07.

National Institutes of Health, U.S. Department of Health and Human Services. *NIH Publication No. 96-3795.*

Pereira, M.A., et al. 2005. Fast-food habits, weight gain, and insulin resistance (the CARDIA study): 15-year prospective analysis. *Lancet.* Jan. 1-7; 365(9453):36-42.

Shape Up America! 10,000 Steps Program. *www.shapeup.org.*

Stewart, K.J., et al. 2005. Exercise and risk factors associated with metabolic syndrome in older adults. *American Journal of Preventive Medicine.* Jan.; 28(1):9-18.

Chapter 7

Duvernoy, C.S., et al. 2005. Weight changes and obesity predict impaired resting and endothelium-dependent myocardial blood flow in postmenopausal women. *Clinical Cardiology.* Jan.; 28(1):13-18.

Eilat-Adar, S., et al. 2005. Association of intentional changes in body weight with coronary heart disease event rates in overweight subjects who have an additional coronary risk factor. *American Journal of Epidemiology.* Feb. 15; 161(4):352-58.

Goel, M.S., et al. 2004. Obesity among U.S. immigrant subgroups by duration of residence. *Journal of the American Medical Association.* Dec. 15; 292(23):2860-67.

Guiliano, Mireille. 2005. *French Women Don't Get Fat.* Alfred A. Knopf.

Li, X., et al. 2004. Childhood adiposity as a predictor of cardiac mass in adulthood: the Bogalusa Heart Study. *Circulation*. Nov. 30; 110(22):3488-92.

Katz, A. Trans-fatty acids and sudden cardiac death. 2002. *Circulation*. Dec.; 80(6):1521-25.

Ma, Y. 2005. Association between dietary carbohydrates and body weight. *American Journal of Epidemiology*. Feb. 15; 161(4):359-67.

Mozaffarian, D., et al. 2004. Trans fatty acids and systemic inflammation in heart failure. *The American Journal of Clinical Nutrition*. Dec.; 80(6):1521-5.

National Health and Nutrition Examination Survey (NHANES). National Institutes of Health. 1999-2000.

Olshansky, S.J., et al. 2005. A potential decline in life expectancy in the United States in the 21st century. *New England Journal of Medicine*. March 17; 352(11):1138-45.

Pomerleau, M., et al. 2004. Effects of exercise intensity on food intake and appetite in women. *The American Journal of Clinical Nutrition*. Nov.; 80(5):1230-36.

Stender, S., Dyerberg, J. 2004. Influence of trans fatty acids on health. *Annals of Nutritional Metabology*. 48(2):61-66.

Trout, D.L., et al. 2004. Atypically high insulin responses to some foods relate to sugars and satiety. *International Journal of Food Science and Nutrition*. Nov.; 55(7):577-97.

Upritchard, J.E., et al. 2005. Modern fat technology: what is the potential for heart health? *The Proceedings of Nutritional Society*. July; 64(3):379-86.

Ziccardi. P., et al. 2002. Reduction of inflammatory cytokine concentrations and improvement of endothelial functions in obese women after weight loss over one year. *Circuation*. Feb. 19; 105(7):9075-76.

Chapter 8

Albert, C.M., et al. 2005. Phobic anxiety and risk of coronary heart disease and sudden cardiac death among women. *Circulation*. Feb. 1; 111(4):480-87.

Eaker, E.D., et al. 2004. Does job strain increase the risk for coronary heart disease or death in men and women? The Framingham Offspring Study. *American Journal of Epidemiology*. May 15; 159(10):950-58.

Lavie, C.J., Milani, R.V. 2005. Prevalence of hostility in young coronary artery disease patients and effects of cardiac rehabilitation and exercise training. *Mayo Clinic Proceeding*. March; 80(3):335-42.

Koton, S., et al. 2004. Triggering risk factors for ischemic stroke: a case-crossover study. *Neurology*. Dec. 14; 63(11):2006-10.

Matthews, K.A., et al. 2004. Blood pressure reactivity to psychological stress predicts hypertension in the CARDIA study. *Circulation*. July 6; 110(1):74-8.

Sotile, Wayne. M., Ph.D., with Canto-Cooke, Robin. 2003. *Thriving with Heart Disease*. Free Press.

Zauberman, G., Lynch, J.G. Jr. 2005. Resource slack and propensity to discount delayed investments of time versus money. *Journal of Experimental Psychology*. Feb.; 134(1):23-37.

Chapter 9

Barth, J., et al. 2004. Depression as a risk factor in mortality for patients with coronary heart disease. *Psychosomatic Medicine*. Nov.-Dec.; 66(6): 802-13.

Carney, R.M., et al. 2004. Depression as a risk factor for post-MI

mortality. *Journal of the American College of Cardiology*. July 21;
44(2):472.

Moser, D.K., Dracup, K. 2004. Role of spousal anxiety and depression in patients' psychosocial recovery after a cardiac event.
Psychosomatic Medicine. July-Aug.; 66(4):527-32.

O'Connor, C.M., Joynt, K.E. 2004. Depression: are we ignoring an
important comorbidity in heart failure. *Journal of the American
College of Cardiology*. May 5; 43(9):1542-49.

Rozanski, A. 2005. The epidemiology, pathophysiology, and management of psychosocial risk factors in cardiac practice: the emerging
field of behavioral cardiology. *Journal of the American College of
Cardiology*. Mar. 1; 45(5):637-51.

Rutledge, T. et al. 2004. Social networks are associated with lower
mortality rates among women with suspected coronary disease:
the National Heart, Lung, and Blood Institute-Sponsored Women's
Ischemia Syndrome Evaluation study. *Psychosomaic Medicine*. Nov.-
Dec.; 66(6):882-8.

Sotile, Wayne. M., Ph.D., with Canto-Cooke, Robin. 2003. *Thriving
with Heart Disease*. Free Press.

Wagner, J.D. 2002. Reproductive hormones and cardiovascular disease mechanism of action and clinical implications. *American
Journal of Obstetrics and Gynecology*. Sept.; 29(3):475-93.

Wittstein, I.S., et al. 2005. Neurohumoral features of myocardial
stunning due to sudden emotional stress. *New England Journal of
Medicine*. Feb. 10; 352(6):539-48.

Chapter 10

Brooke, R.D., et al. 2004. Air pollution and cardiovascular disease: a
statement for healthcare professionals from the Expert Panel on

Population and Prevention Science of the American Heart Association. *Circulation.* June 1; 109(21):2655-71.

Desvarieux, M., et al. 2005. Periodontal microbiota and carotid intima-media thickness: the Oral Infections and Vascular Disease Epidemiology Study (INVEST). *Circulation.* Feb. 8; 111(5):576-82.

Frost, L., Vestergaard, P. 2005. Caffeine and risk of atrial fibrillation or flutter: the Danish Diet, Cancer, and Health Study. *The American Journal of Clinical Nutrition.* March; 81(3):578-82.

Gilmour, P., et al. 2005. The procoagulant potential of environmental particles (PM10). *Occupational and Environmental Medicine.* March; 62(3):164-71.

Haas, D.C., et al. 2005. Age-dependent associations between sleep-disordered breathing and hypertension: importance of discriminating between systolic/diastolic hypertension and isolated systolic hypertension in the Sleep Heart Health Study. *Circulation.* Feb. 8; 111(5):576-82.

Kawachi, I. 2005. More evidence on the risks of passive smoking. *British Medical Journal.* Feb. 5; 330(7486):265-6.

Kunzli, N., et al. 2005. Ambient air pollution and atherosclerosis in Los Angeles. *Environmental Health Perspective.* Feb.; 113(2):201-6.

Lee, S., et al. 2003. Caregiving to children and grandchildren and risk of coronary heart disease in women. *American Journal of Public Health.* Nov.; 93(11):1939-44.

Levy, D.T., et al. 2004. Recent trends in home and work smoking bans. *Tobacco Control.* Sept.; 13(3):258-63.

Marcuccio, E., et al. 2003. A survey of attitudes and experiences of women with heart disease. *Women's Health Issues.* Jan.-Feb.; 13(1):23-31.

Montebugnoli, L., Prati, C. 2002. Circulatory dynamics during dental extractions in normal, cardiac and transplant patients. *Journal of the American Dental Association.* April; 133(4):468-72.

Mukamal, K.J., et al. 2004. Caffeinated coffee consumption and mortality after acute myocardial infarction. *American Heart Journal.* June; 147(6):999-1004.

Robertson, R.M. 2001. Women and cardiovascular disease: the risks of misperception and the need for action. *Circulation.* May 15; 103(19):2318-20.

Ruidavets, J.B. 2005. Ozone air pollution is associated with acute myocardial infarction. *Circulation.* Feb., 8; 111(5):563-69.

Sandhu, R.S., et al. 2005. C-reactive protein, and coronary artery disease. *Inhalation Toxicology.* June-July; (7-8):409-13.

Taheri, S., et al. 2004. Short sleep duration is associated with reduced leptin, elevated ghrelin, and increased body mass index. *Public Library of Science Medicine.* Dec.; 1(3):e62.

Vorona, R.D., et al. 2005. Overweight and obese patients in a primary care population report less sleep than patients with a normal body mass index. *Archives of Internal Medicine.* Jan. 10; 165(1):15-16.

Woodward, A., et al. 2004. Deaths caused by secondhand smoke: estimates are consistent. *Tobacco Control.* Sept.; 13(3):319-20.

Zhang, X., et al. 2005. Association of passive smoking by husbands with prevalence of stroke among Chinese women nonsmokers. *American Journal of Epidemiology.* Feb. 1; 161(3):213-8.

Index

A

abdominal fat
  benefits of exercise, 139
  measurement and ratio, 37
  in metabolic syndrome, 42
  as risk factor, 37, 39, 157
  See also overweight and obesity
activity. *See* exercise
alcohol. *See* wine
All Heart Vinaigrette, 73
almonds, 77
anger and hostility, 204–7
angiography, 24
anthocyanins, 110–13
antioxidants, 108
  See also phytonutrients; poly-
    phenols
anxiety. *See* emotional issues
aromatherapy, 192–93, 230
  Blissful Office Blend mist, 196
asparagus, 126–27
avocados, 131
  in Guacamole, 133

B

baths, 230–32, 233
beans
  in Chili con Kathy, 93
  effect on cholesterol and tri-
    glyceride levels, 91
  in Meatless Cassoulet, 98–99

  soy, 101–4
  varieties and preparations, 92–94
beer, 60
berries
  Berry Fruity Chutney, 116
  blueberries, 111–12
  cranberries, 115–17
  raspberries, 113–15
  strawberries, 113
beta-carotene, 113, 123
Blissful Office Blend, 196
blood lipids. *See entries beginning with*
  cholesterol; triglycerides
blood pressure, dietary influences
  folate, 118
  onions, 121
  oranges, 131
  salt, 102
  spinach, 127
  vegetarian diet, 100–101
  whole grains, 96
blood pressure, high
  danger of, 29, 41–43, 50
  in metabolic syndrome, 42
  monitoring, 43–44
blood pressure, nondietary
  influences
    depression, 204
    exercise, 138
    forgiveness of grudges, 208
    meditation, 193